Treatment of Ongoing Hemorrhage

Chad G. Ball • Elijah Dixon
Editors

Treatment of Ongoing Hemorrhage

The Art and Craft of Stopping Severe Bleeding

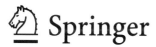 Springer

Editors
Chad G. Ball, MD
Hepatobiliary and Pancreatic Surgery
Trauma and Acute Care Surgery
University of Calgary
Foothills Medical Centre
Calgary, AB, Canada

Elijah Dixon, MD
Hepatobiliary and Pancreatic Surgery
Division of General Surgery
Faculty of Medicine
Foothills Medical Centre
Calgary, AB, Canada

ISBN 978-3-319-87571-2   ISBN 978-3-319-63495-1   (eBook)
DOI 10.1007/978-3-319-63495-1

Printed on acid-free paper

This Springer imprint is published by Springer Nature
The registered company is Springer International Publishing AG
The registered company address is: Gewerbestrasse 11, 6330 Cham, Switzerland

Preface

Persistent life-threatening hemorrhage remains amongst the most feared scenarios for every practicing clinician. "Bleeding to death" is not only the most common etiology of trauma mortality on earth but also the most frequent cause of a physician's sleepless nights. Whether ongoing bleeding occurs within the operating theater during an elective resection at a quaternary referral center, an emergency department in a remote rural hospital, and an endoscopy suite in a medium-sized center or on the battlefield in a far forward extreme and hostile environment, persistent hemorrhage could easily be described as our utmost acute challenge in medicine.

The aim of the textbook is to provide the reader with a "no-nonsense," salient, practical, and experience-based summary of technical solutions for stopping massive ongoing hemorrhage prior to the demise of our patients. Each chapter directly addresses a unique area or scenario and is authored by impressively all-star experienced clinicians who share their best and most eloquent technical solutions to the issue of arresting persistent life-threatening hemorrhage. While individual authors are always credited with a specific chapter, each contributor acknowledges that in many cases, these tricks have been handed down from clinician to clinician beginning prior to the practice of Hippocrates. Stopping ongoing bleeding in an efficient and smooth manner is something that separates the master clinician from the one who is still growing. It is also amongst the most impressive things to watch amongst our colleagues.

We hope this textbook will serve as a tremendous technical resource the next time you are faced with caring for a persistently bleeding patient nearing physiologic extremis.

Calgary, AB, Canada

Chad G. Ball
Elijah Dixon

Acknowledgments

Chad G. Ball I would like to thank my children (Sydney, Griffin, and Riley) most of all for filling my life with joy. I would also like to thank my partner Elijah Dixon for his continued support and an amazing journey together. Finally, the drive and vision to create this textbook would not have been possible without the endless advice, superb training, and deep friendship from all of my surgical mentors (Keith Lillemoe, David Feliciano, Thomas Howard, Andrew Nicol, Pradeep Navsaria, Morad Hameed, Henry Pitt, Attila Nakeeb, Grace Rozycki, Jeffrey Nicholas, Christopher Dente, Amy Wyrzykowski, Michael House, Nicholas Zyromski, Joseph Tector, Paul Greig, Fred Brenneman, Andrew Kirkpatrick, Francis Sutherland, Bryce Taylor, Bernard Langer, Gary Vercruysse, Peter Rhee, Kenji Inaba, Gene Moore, Chistopher Doig, and Neil Parry).

Elijah Dixon I would like to thank my family for their support over the years – my daughters Natalie May Dixon and Gabrielle Dawn Dixon who put up with my crazy hours and my parents Donald Dixon and Jamie Nelson-Dixon. I would like to thank my partner Dr. Chad Ball who is the driving force behind this exciting new book.

Contents

Contributors

Chad G. Ball, MD Hepatobiliary and Pancreatic Surgery, Trauma and Acute Care Surgery, University of Calgary, Foothills Medical Centre, Calgary, AB, Canada

Kristofer M. Charlton-Ouw, MD, FACS Department of Cardiothoracic and Vascular Surgery, Memorial Hermann Heart & Vascular Institute at Texas Medical Center, Houston, TX, USA

Clay Cothren Burlew, MD, FACS Department of Surgery, Denver Health Medical Center and University of Colorado School of Medicine, Denver, CO, USA

Martin A. Croce, MD Department of Surgery, University of Tennessee Health Science Center, Memphis, TN, USA

Elijah Dixon, MD Hepatobiliary and Pancreatic Surgery, Division of General Surgery, Faculty of Medicine, Foothills Medical Centre, Calgary, AB, Canada

Joseph J. DuBose, MD, FACS, FCCM Department of Surgery, Uniformed Services University of the Health Sciences, University of California, Davis, CA, USA

David V. Feliciano, MD Battersby Professor Emeritus, Indiana University School of Medicine, Indianapolis, IN, USA

University of Maryland School of Medicine, Shock Trauma Center, Baltimore, MD, USA

Charles Fox, MD Department of Surgery, Denver Health Medical Center and University of Colorado School of Medicine, Denver, CO, USA

Scott Gmora, MD, FRCSC, FACS General/Bariatric Surgery, St. Joseph's Healthcare, Mcmaster University, Hamilton, ON, Canada

Sean C. Grondin, MD, FRCSC, MPH, FACS Department of Surgery, University of Calgary, Calgary, AB, Canada

Morad Hameed, MD, MPH, FRCSC, FACS Department of Surgery, University of British Columbia, Vancouver, BC, Canada

Alan W. Hemming, MD, MSc Department of Surgery, University of California San Diego, La Jolla, CA, USA

Kenji Inaba, MD Division of Trauma & Critical Care, LAC+USC Medical Center, Los Angeles, CA, USA

Andrew W. Kirkpatrick, MD, MHSc, FRCSC, FACS Departments of Surgery and Critical Care Medicine, Foothills Hospital, Calgary, AB, Canada

Stefan W. Leichtle, MD Division of Acute Care Surgical Services, Virginia Commonwealth University Medical Center, Richmond, VA, USA

Keith D. Lillemoe, MD Department of Surgery, Massachusetts General Hospital, Boston, MA, USA

Nathan R. Manley, MD, MPH Department of Surgery, University of Tennessee Health Science Center, Memphis, TN, USA

Paul B. Mcbeth, MD Departments of Critical Care Medicine and Surgery, University of Calgary, Calgary, AB, Canada

Kristin L. Mekeel, MD Department of Surgery, University of California San Diego, La Jolla, CA, USA

Rachid Mohamed, MD, FRCPC Therapeutic Endoscopy, Peter Lougheed Centre, Calgary, AB, Canada

Ernest E. Moore, MD Department of Surgery, Denver Health Medical Center and University of Colorado School of Medicine, Denver, CO, USA

Pradeep Navsaria, MBChB, MMed(Surgery), FCS(SA), FACS Department of Surgery, Trauma, Groote Schuur Hospital and University of Cape Town, Observatory, Western Cape, South Africa

Andrew John Nicol, MBChB, FCS (SA), PhD Department of Surgery, Trauma, Groote Schuur Hospital and University of Cape Town, Observatory, Western Cape, South Africa

Neil G. Parry, MD, FRCSC, BSc General Surgery, Trauma and Critical Care, Departments of Surgery and Medicine, Schulich School of Medicine, Western University, London, ON, Canada

Madhukar S. Patel, MD, MBA, ScM General Surgery, Massachusetts General Hospital, Boston, MA, USA

Colin Schieman, BSc, MD, FRCSC Department of Surgery, University of Calgary, Calgary, AB, Canada

Parsia A. Vagefi, MD, FACS Liver Transplantation, Massachusetts General Hospital, Boston, MA, USA

Jason K. Wong, MD, FRCPC Division of Interventional Radiology, Department of Diagnostic Imaging, Foothills Medical Centre, Calgary, AB, Canada

Chapter 1
Medical Principles of Hemostasis: Just Give Me the Nuts and Bolts!

Paul B. McBeth

Case Scenario

A 73-year-old male involved in a pedestrian versus motor vehicle collision is critically injured (pelvic fracture, splenic and liver lacerations, traumatic brain injury, and open femur fracture). Hypotension takes you to the operating room where you engage in a damage control procedure. Despite stopping all major vessel/organ hemorrhage, your patient continues the dreaded "ooze" from all sites. He's well into the third cycle of his massive transfusion (protocol), but it seems to be ineffective!…

Introduction

In this chapter, we outline the general medical principles of hemostasis. The surgical focus of a patient with ongoing hemorrhage is to stop bleeding. This may take the form of an open surgical procedure or a catheter-directed approach by an interventional radiologist. In the heat of the moment, you're unlikely to be thinking about details of the coagulation cascade or the differential diagnosis of a particular thromboelastogram. In trauma patients with active hemorrhage, the key is recognizing the injury pattern and the degree of physiologic derangement, followed by prompt execution of targeted resuscitation with definitive surgical management. The purpose of this chapter is to provide an overview of the practical points in the medical management of an actively bleeding patient.

P.B. McBeth (✉)
Departments of Critical Care Medicine and Surgery, University of Calgary,
Calgary, AB, Canada
e-mail: pmcbeth@gmail.com

© Springer International Publishing AG 2018   1
C.G. Ball, E. Dixon (eds.), *Treatment of Ongoing Hemorrhage*,
DOI 10.1007/978-3-319-63495-1_1

Fig. 1.1 Triad of death

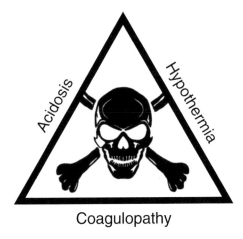

Coagulopathy

Damage Control Resuscitation

Principles of damage control resuscitation (DCR) have evolved over the past 10 years based on experience with recent international armed conflicts and our improved understanding of trauma-associated coagulopathy (TAC). The foundations of DCR are damage control surgery along with permissive hypotension and hemostatic resuscitation. This systematic approach is targeted at maintaining adequate circulating volume with early correction of acidosis, hypothermia, coagulopathy, and hypoperfusion (Fig. 1.1). It begins in the prehospital setting, followed by the emergency department and continues through to the operating room (OR) and intensive care unit (ICU) (Fig. 1.2).

Injury Pattern Recognition

Understanding and recognizing the pattern of injury are essential for early execution of targeted management of the critically ill trauma patient. This skill is acquired from extensive time spent at the bedside resuscitating trauma patients. Early recognition of injury patterns and targeted interventions are needed to correct acute physiologic derangements. For example, patients in extremis need urgent evaluation to rule out nonhemorrhagic causes of shock, such as tension pneumothorax and pericardial tamponade. Not all patients require DCR, but this early recognition of physiological derangement is essential to initiate early interventions. Key triggers of DCR are outlined in Table 1.1.

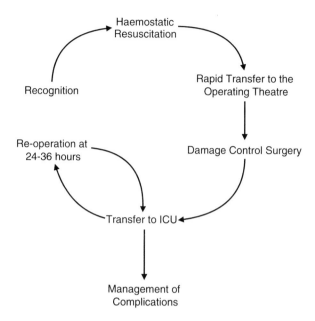

Fig. 1.2 Stages of damage control resuscitation

Table 1.1 Triggers of DCR

Parameter	Value
Systolic blood pressure	<90 mmHg
Temperature	<36 °C
pH	<7.2
Base deficit	> −6
Hgb	<90 g/L
INR	>1.5

Permissive Hypotension

The primary goal in management of hemorrhagic shock is to control blood loss. Permissive hypotension, however, is a temporary strategy to limit fluid therapy prior to surgical control of hemorrhage. This can be achieved by either delayed initiation or limited volume of fluids given. The purpose is to minimize dilutional coagulopathy and hypothermia from excessive fluid administration. Overzealous fluid resuscitation to maintain a normal blood pressure may also result in the displacement of an established clot. It is postulated that maintaining a lower systolic blood pressure target of around 80 mmHg may reduce this risk. At present, there is evolving evidence to support the practice of permissive hypotension. The exception to this rule is in patients with suspected traumatic brain injury (TBI) .

Hemostatic Resuscitation

Hemostatic resuscitation has become a dominant aspect of damage control resuscitation. This resuscitation technique aims to deliver blood components to resemble whole blood and forms the basis of most massive transfusion protocols. Fresh whole blood (FWB) is considered the optimum transfusion product in patients with massive hemorrhage because of its physiologic properties [1]. For a variety of reasons including availability, storage limitations, and infection disease risk, FWB is not available in civilian trauma care systems.

The goal of hemostatic resuscitation is to administer blood components in a ratio that resembles whole blood and to limit the complications of aggressive crystalloid fluid resuscitation. This can be achieved by a resuscitation strategy aimed to provide a balanced transfusion delivery of pRBC, FFP, and platelets with a ratio of 1:1:1 [2]. Other adjuncts to support clot formation and stabilization include administration of calcium and tranexamic acid (TXA). There is growing interest in using prothrombin complex concentrate (PCC) and fibrinogen concentrate in patients with massive hemorrhage as an alternative to FFP and cryoprecipitate. The advantages are low volume, standard dosing, reduced viral transmission risk, and fewer transfusion reactions.

Temperature

Trauma patients presenting with hypothermia are at risk of hypothermia-induced coagulopathy and worse outcomes. Aggressive rewarming attempts of hypothermic patients begin in the prehospital setting. Prevention of heat loss and active rewarming should be provided to patients with long prehospital transport times. Preheating of the trauma bay is essential. You and your colleagues will be uncomfortable with the room temperature, but it is a key factor for prevention of further cooling of the patient. As an adjunct to the primary survey, all clothing should be removed from the patient and replaced with preheated blankets or a forced-air warming device. Patients with severe hypothermia may require extreme techniques including extracorporeal support.

Damage Control Surgery

The principle of damage control surgery (DCS) is to prioritize the physiological and biochemical stabilization of a patient rather than providing definitive repair of all injuries [3]. The purpose of DCS is to identify and stop sources of surgically correctable hemorrhage and to control contamination. The surgery or procedure should be directed to achieve these goals. This is not the time for pontification. You need to be efficient, direct, and purposeful with your movements. Your focus should be on hemostatic maneuvers such as vessel ligation or temporary shunting. Avoid extensive vascular repairs or grafting. Use laparotomy packs to control diffuse bleeding such as liver lacerations. Be mindful of time—a DCS should take less than an hour. Anything more is compromising the patient. Clear communication with your anesthesia team regarding the degree of injury and perioperative plan is essential. Early mobilization of supporting teams for angiographic embolization, ICU, and CT should be considered. Efficient and directed surgical intervention is needed for a favorable outcome. Don't delay transfer to the ICU by closing fascia. Apply a temporary abdominal closure and get out early. Once complete, the patient should be transferred to the ICU for further management and correction of physiological derangement.

Postoperative Management (Intensive Care Unit)

Once the patient arrives in the ICU, your focus will shift to initiate secondary resuscitation in an effort to rewarm and correct the patient's acidosis and coagulopathy. Efforts to maintain adequate oxygen delivery are required and facilitated by optimized ventilation techniques and intravascular volume resuscitation. Your goal is to restore near-normal physiology through restoration of intravascular volume and normothermia and correction of the patient's coagulopathy. Once these goals are achieved, the patient is then safe to return to the OR for re-exploration and definitive management. Lastly, a complete physical exam and careful review of diagnostic imaging are mandatory to identify and document all injuries. Missed injuries are common and all trauma needs to be identified.

Ventilation

Early management of ventilation in the ICU is targeted to ensure optimal gas exchange and to avoid further lung injury. Given the large volume resuscitation your patient has just received, they are at risk of developing acute respiratory distress syndrome (ARDS). Massive resuscitation leads to decreased compliance of the lungs. The same effect is seen with decreased extrathoracic lung compliance from increased abdominal pressure and chest wall edema. The initial mode of ventilation should be set at pressure-regulated volume control with a tidal volume of 6–8 mL/kg. Peak inspiratory pressure should be limited to less than 40 mmHg. The FiO_2 should be initially set at 100% and titrated to maintain oxygenation saturation of 92% or greater. The positive end-expiratory pressure (PEEP) is initially set at 5 cm H_2O and titrated upward in increments of 2 cm H_2O to allow downward titration of the FiO_2. Be mindful of cardiac function as high PEEP will impede venous return to the heart. Patients with worsening oxygenation may require full sedation and paralysis to optimize ventilation. If oxygenation continues to be a challenge, the inspiration to expiration (I/E) ratio should be reduced. Prone positioning will often improve oxygenation by recruiting anterior gas exchange units, but this is often impractical in patients with an open abdomen. Other advanced therapies include high-frequency oscillating ventilation (HFOV) and ECMO. Recent data suggest HFOV causes increased harm. The use of ECMO often requires full anticoagulation which is impractical in the majority of trauma patients with significant tissue injury and bleeding risk.

Resuscitation

Appropriate vascular access is needed in the secondary resuscitation phase. Lines placed prehospital or in the emergency department should be replaced using sterile technique. Internal jugular or subclavian central venous access should also be achieved.

Postoperative resuscitation is targeted to maintain ongoing hemostasis and to ensure adequate end-organ perfusion. To achieve this, intravascular volume resuscitation should be guided by adequate urinary output, restoration of vital signs, clearance of lactate, normalization of base deficit, and achievement of a central venous gas oxygen saturation ($ScvO_2$) between 68% and 72%. Initial fluid selection should aim to correct any underlying coagulopathy. Now is the time to demonstrate your skills of data interpretation from thromboelastography (see TEG section). Monitor Hgb levels for signs of ongoing bleeding. Avoid excessive use of crystalloids as this may lead to increased tissue edema, with resulting compartment syndrome, and worsening coagulopathy. Additional tools to assess cardiac function include pulmonary artery catheterization, PiCCO catheter, and focused beside transthoracic or transesophageal echocardiography.

Rewarming

Active rewarming is an essential aspect of ongoing resuscitation. To facilitate optimal rewarming, the ICU room should be preheated to 30 °C. Once the patient arrives to the ICU any wet linen should be removed and skin dried off. A forced-air warming device is used to cover the patient and set to 40 °C. All infusion lines and the ventilator circuit should be equipped with warming devices. Your goal is to warm the patient to 37 °C within 6 h of arrival to the ICU. If a patient has not rewarmed appropriately, then other techniques may include pleural lavage with warm saline using chest tubes and intravenous warming catheters. In patients with temperatures less than 32 °C, consideration of extracorporeal rewarming with ECMO is needed.

Correction of Acidosis

With rewarming and fluid resuscitation, a patient's metabolism will revert from anaerobic to aerobic. This, combined with the clearance of lactate, results in the self-correction of acidosis. The administration of sodium bicarbonate is often unnecessary.

Return to Operating Theater

Once the physiologic derangements have resolved, the patient should return to the operating room as soon as possible for re-exploration, definitive repair, and attempted wound closure. The process starts with the removal of the temporary abdominal closure and intra-abdominal packs. This is followed by a complete evaluation of intra-abdominal organs to identify the temporized primary injuries and to evaluate for any unrecognized injuries. Once this is complete, then proceed with definitive repair. Be sure to anticipate potential complications, and consider failure modes of your repair (fail-safe repair). Complication rates are often higher in DCS patients. Patients with significant injury and resuscitation may go on to develop significant bowel wall edema. This will worsen with time and has the potential to cause intra-abdominal hypertension and potential abdominal compartment syndrome. If you are unable to close the abdominal wall, then a temporary abdominal closure may be reapplied. Remember, your goal should be to close the abdominal wall on this admission to hospital. This may require repeated trips to the OR for further washout and abdominal wall tightening. Closure of the abdominal wall is directly proportional to surgeon effort.

Coagulopathy

Uncontrollable hemorrhage is responsible for 30–40% of trauma mortality and accounts for almost 50% of deaths occurring in the initial 24 h following the traumatic incident. Trauma-induced coagulopathy has been identified as the most common preventable cause of post-injury mortality and remains the main challenge for improved outcome in this critically injured cohort [5]. On admission, 25–35% of trauma patients present with coagulopathy, which is associated with a sevenfold increase in morbidity and mortality.

The mechanisms of acute traumatic coagulopathy are multifactorial and involve various elements of the coagulation system. The primary mechanism is the uncontrolled release of tissue factor from endothelial injury. This leads to increased thrombin generation and consumption of clotting factors. Other factors also include platelet dysfunction and activation of fibrinolytic pathways. The combination of these is worsened by acidosis, hypothermia, and hypoperfusion.

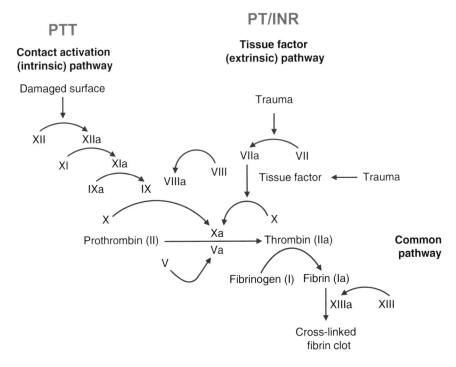

Fig. 1.3 The classic model of the coagulation cascade

Practically, at the bedside, the two most important clinical factors contributing to acute traumatic coagulopathy are the degree of tissue injury and tissue hypoperfusion. Other important contributing factors include hemodilution, hypothermia, acidosis, systemic inflammation, and genetics. Altogether, these contribute to the bloody vicious cycle.

Standard measurements of coagulopathy have historically been based on prothrombin time (PT), partial thromboplastin time (PTT), and international normalized ratio (INR). The PT and PTT measure the extrinsic and intrinsic clotting pathway functions, respectively. The classical model of the coagulation cascade is shown in Fig. 1.3. Although the classic model of coagulation is academically interesting, practically it has very little relevance in clinical trauma care. This model has recently been challenged by the cell-based model of coagulation which describes coagulation in three overlapping stages: initiation, amplification, and propagation of clotting. This model gives a clearer picture of in vivo coagulation function. The diagnosis of traumatic coagulopathy has historically been made if PTT or PT were prolonged by more than 1.5 times the upper limit of normal [4]. These traditional measures of hemostasis do not accurately describe the nature of the coagulopathy of trauma. They lack the ability to identify specific coagulation factor deficiencies and are unable to provide real-time monitoring of coagulation defects. More recently, thromboelastography (TEG) has been incorporated into trauma care as a tool for the analysis of several aspects of clot formation and strength [6, 7].

Fig. 1.4 TEG sample processing

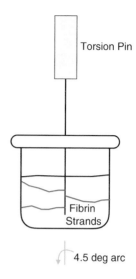

TEG

Our understanding of mechanisms and pathophysiology of TAC has improved dramatically over the past 10 years. As such, the integration of viscoelastic coagulation assays (VCA) has become a useful adjunct in guiding hemostatic therapy in clinical situations of massive hemorrhage and coagulopathy. Unlike conventional clotting tests, VCA provides a functional measure of the entire clotting cascade including the extrinsic and intrinsic pathways. This evaluation method provides a dynamic characterization of the coagulation system through the evaluation of clotting time, clot formation, clot stability, and fibrinolysis [7]. VCA is also used to identify the speed of initial fibrin formation (fibrin burst), the influence of clotting factors and anticoagulants, measures of platelet and fibrinogen levels, and clot firmness. Based on these results, specific hemostatic abnormalities can be identified, thereby providing a tool for individualizing transfusion resuscitation and coagulation management. Goal-directed therapy targeted at specific coagulation defects results in the use of fewer blood products, therefore limiting a patient's exposure to transfusion side effects. This targeted approach has the potential to improve patient outcomes and reduce cost.

Originally described by Hartert in 1948 [8], thromboelastography (TEG) is currently widely used as a point-of-care tool to detect TAC by evaluation of a patient's coagulation state. It is used to identify the viscoelastic properties of a sample of whole blood and relies on a small volume (0.3 ml) of blood placed into a sample cup (Fig. 1.4). Within this cup a pin is suspended by a torsion wire. The cup is then oscillated to simulate venous flow. As the blood begins to clot, strands of platelets and fibrin will couple the cup to the pin. This coupling effect will grow as further clot is formed resulting in the transmission of torque from the oscillating cup to the torsion wire. The peaks of these recorded oscillations are used to create a TEG profile as

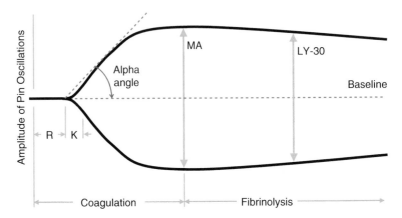

Fig. 1.5 TEG tracing

Fig. 1.6 Sample of TEG tracings

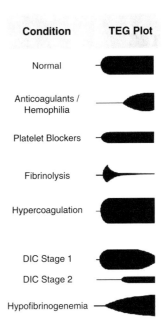

shown in Fig. 1.5. Using computer software, the TEG plot is presented along with a series of measured and calculated values (Table 1.2). This quantitative and qualitative evaluation of viscoelastic behavior of blood can be used to identify the pattern of coagulopathy (Fig. 1.6).

Practically, VCA can be used to guide resuscitation of a trauma patient by identifying specific coagulation defects and the need for massive transfusion. As a point-of-care tool, initial VCA results are available within 10–20 min to help guide

Table 1.2 TEG values and interpretation

Parameter		Normal range	Description	Measures

Clotting time	R	5.0–10.0 min	Represents the enzymatic reaction
			Time the analyzer is started until initial fibrin formation (TEG reaches a 2 mm amplitude)
			Rate of thromboplastin generation
			Intrinsic pathway function (factors XII, XI, and VIII)
			Elongated R
			  Coagulation factor deficiencies
			  Anticoagulant drugs (warfarin, heparin)
			Short R
			  Presence of hypercoagulability
				Clotting factors (intrinsic pathway)

Clot kinetics	K	1.0–3.0 min	Represents the speed of clot formation Time from the end of R until the clot reaches 20 mm Rate at which a relatively firm clot is formed Function of the intrinsic pathway, platelets, and fibrinogen Platelet activity reaches its peak and fibrinogen activity is prolonged if there is coagulation factor deficiency or platelet-inhibiting drugs Short K Increased platelet activity	Fibrinogen, platelet number

	Alpha	53.0–72.0°	The alpha angle is calculated by taking the tangent of the curve produced to reach the K value
			Angle created by the R arm and the K inclination
			Rate at which a solid clot is formed
			Indicator of the quality of platelets and fibrinogen
			High angle
			  Higher platelet activity or blood fibrinogen
			Low angle
			  Anticoagulants are or platelet inhibitors are present
				Fibrinogen, platelet number

(continued)

Table 1.2 (continued)

Parameter		Normal range	Description	Measures

Clot strength	MA	50.0–70.0 mm	Maximum amplitude
			Measure of the strength of the clot
			The greatest diameter of the clot and a measure of the clot's elasticity
			High MA
			  Higher quality of platelet, fibrinogen, and factor XIII. Relies on the interaction of fibrin and platelets
			Low MA
			  Insufficient platelet-fibrin clot formation
				Platelet number and function

	G	5.3–12.4 dynes/cm^2	Calculated value of clot strength It is a part of the maximum amplitude Obtained with the following formula: 5000 MA/(100 − MA) Indicator of how firm the clot is Very sensitive to changes in maximum amplitude	Entire coagulation cascade

Coagulation index	CI	−3 to +3	It is a numerical value that may be positive or negative, ranging from −3 to +3
			Low CI
			  Suggestive of hypocoagulation
			High CI
			  Suggestive of hypercoagulation
				Entire coagulation cascade

Clot stability	LY30	0–3%	Measure of fibrinolysis Time interval between MA and 0 amplitude in the TEG	Fibrinolysis

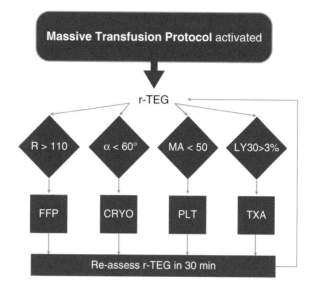

Fig. 1.7 Massive transfusion protocol incorporating TEG (Adapted from Moore EE, et al.)

patient-specific resuscitation strategies. Compared with routine coagulation tests, VCA can also detect the anticoagulant effect of severe metabolic derangements such as acidosis and hypothermia.

The following table outlines TEG values obtained from a blood sample. See Table 1.1. Although these values can sometimes be overwhelming to interpret, a few simple steps can be used to help guide your resuscitation. Incorporation of these rules into a transfusion protocol may also be helpful. All patients presenting with a significant injury should have a VCA drawn as part of their initial trauma bloodwork. This also includes any patients requiring massive transfusion for active hemorrhage. Diagnosis and treatment algorithms incorporating VCA analysis for bleeding patients have been developed. The following flow diagram is based on the work of Moore et al. [9] and has not been evaluated in a prospective randomized trial (Fig. 1.7). Once a correction has been made, a reassessment VCA should be repeated 30 min after administration of coagulation factors or blood products to help guide further management.

Understanding Fibrinolysis

Fibrinolysis is an important contributor to trauma-induced coagulopathy. To counter the adverse effects of excessive fibrinolysis, tranexamic acid (TXA) has been demonstrated to reduce transfusion requirements and improve mortality in trauma patients. As our understanding of fibrinolysis expands and our ability to characterize it using VCA improves, antifibrinolytic treatments may become tailored to patient-specific needs. Recent data published identified three distinct fibrinolytic phenotypes (hyperfibrinolysis, physiologic, and hypofibrinolysis (shutdown)) supporting the need for further study and the suggestion of a patient-specific approach to TXA administration [10]. The authors suggest the characterization of fibrinolysis greater than 3% should be the trigger for antifibrinolytic therapy.

In the end, damage control resuscitation and principles of hemostasis go hand in hand. By offering a structured, efficient, and timely combination of the therapies described in this chapter, your critically bleeding patient will have a much improved chance of life over death.

> I would like to see the day when somebody is appointed surgeon who has no hands, for the operative part is the least part of the work. Harvey W. Cushing.

Take-Home Points
1. Damage control resuscitation (DCR) is a resuscitation strategy based on damage control surgery along with permissive hypotension and hemostatic resuscitation.
2. Hemostatic resuscitation is a strategy aimed at delivering blood components to resemble whole blood and forms the basis of most massive transfusion protocols.
3. Early correction of metabolic and physiologic derangements is essential to improve patient survival.
4. The etiology of trauma-associated coagulopathy is multiple factorial but primarily driven by degree of tissue injury and tissue hypoxia.
5. The thromboelastogram provides detailed information regarding the dynamics of in vivo whole blood clot formation and can be used to identify specific clotting function abnormalities including degree of fibrinolytic activity.

> *I would like to see the day when somebody is appointed surgeon who has no hands, for the operative part is the least part of the work.* Harvey W. Cushing

References

1. Holcomb JB, del Junco DJ, Fox EE, et al. The prospective, observational, multicenter, major trauma transfusion (PROMMTT) study: comparative effectiveness of a time-varying treatment with competing risks. JAMA Surg. 2013;148(2):127–36.
2. Holcomb JB, Tilley BC, Baraniuk S, et al. Transfusion of plasma, platelets, and red blood cells in a 1:1:1 vs a 1:1:2 ratio and mortality in patients with severe trauma: the PROPPR randomized clinical trial. JAMA. 2015;313(5):471–82.
3. Ball CG. Damage control surgery. Curr Opin Crit Care. 2015 Dec;21(6):538–43.
4. Stainsby D, MacLennan S, Thomas D, Isaac J, Hamilton PJ. Guidelines on the management of massive blood loss. Br J Haematol. 2006;135:634–41.
5. Palmer L, Martin L. Traumatic coagulopathy—part 1: pathophysiology and diagnosis. J Vet Emerg Crit Care (San Antonio). 2014;24:63–74.
6. Wozniak D, Adamik B. Thromboelastography. Anestezjol Intens Ter. 2011;43:244–7.
7. Kashuk JL, Moore EE, Sawyer M, Wohlauer M, Pezold M, Barnett C, et al. Primary fibrinolysis is integral in the pathogenesis of the acute coagulopathy of trauma. Ann Surg. 2010; 252:434–44.
8. Hartert H. Blutgerinnungsstudien mit der Thrombelastographie, einem neuen Untersuchungsvefahren. Klin Wochenschr. 1948;26:577–83.

9. Pezold M, Moore EE, Wohlauer M, Sauaia A, Gonzalez E, Banerjee A, Silliman CC. Viscoelastic clot strength predicts coagulation-related mortality within 15 minutes. Surgery. 2012 Jan;151(1):48–54.
10. Moore HB, Moore EE, Gonzalez E, Chapman MP, Chin TL, Silliman CC, Banerjee A, Sauaia A. Hyperfibrinolysis, physiologic fibrinolysis, and fibrinolysis shutdown: the spectrum of postinjury fibrinolysis and relevance to antifibrinolytic therapy. J Trauma Acute Care Surg. 2014 Dec;77(6):811–7.

Chapter 2
Surgical Principles of Hemostasis: Ideas Worth Considering

Elijah Dixon and Chad G. Ball

Case Scenario

A 21-year-old female is crushed between a wall and a large delivery truck. She presents with catastrophic ongoing hemorrhage from nearly all of her intra-abdominal organs and will require your absolute best to successfully get her to the ICU after the operative procedure…

The first and foremost priority for any surgeon dealing with bleeding is to control the situation, convey calm focus to the team, and direct all energy toward working the problem. Remember that you are a SURGEON! You have trained for years to be an expert in the control of bleeding. There is no one more qualified than you in the room to deal with bleeding! Few careers involve the depth and length of training that we get in surgery; consequently the surgeon should be expert at controlling his environment to achieve his goal. Loss of control, decompensation of demeanor, getting angry, yelling, and generally creating an environment of anxiety for the other team members all represent failures by the surgeon to use the heightened energy that is often generated in the setting of poorly controlled bleeding toward resolution and control of the problem. You are a highly trained professional at the top of your game and the top of the healthcare team hierarchy – *YOU ARE A SURGEON. ACT LIKE ONE!*

Bleeding is only a problem for the unprepared surgeon. Division of the aorta, vena cava, or middle hepatic vein is straightforward to control and repair when it is easily accessible, and the surgeon is prepared for it. A middle hepatic vein partially torn in a large obese male with a small incision and a surgeon poorly prepared can

E. Dixon (✉)

Hepatobiliary and Pancreatic Surgery, Division of General Surgery, Faculty of Medicine, Foothills Medical Centre, Calgary, AB, Canada

e-mail: Elijah.Dixon@albertahealthservices.ca

C.G. Ball

Hepatobiliary and Pancreatic Surgery, Trauma and Acute Care Surgery, University of Calgary, Foothills Medical Centre, Calgary, AB, Canada

© Springer International Publishing AG 2018

C.G. Ball, E. Dixon (eds.), *Treatment of Ongoing Hemorrhage*,

DOI 10.1007/978-3-319-63495-1_2

be life-threatening. All possible problems should be anticipated BEFORE the operation. If the surgeon has mentally planned out what he/she will do in different situations, they are calm when it happens and able to deal with it. It's very similar to the elite athlete visualizing key parts of the game or the fight – it becomes self-fulfilling if and when they encounter that situation. Just like athletics, for the well-prepared surgeon, time will often slow down during a "crisis" (as opposed to speed up). *VISUALIZE AND PREPARE FOR ALL SCENARIOS LIKE AN ELITE ATHLETE – YOU ARE A SURGEON.*

Almost all scenarios involving very significant bleeding can benefit from an improvement in exposure. While you plan to act on your preoperative visualizations of this particular bleeding scenario, improve your exposure. This alone will often be all that is needed to convert poorly controlled bleeding to easily dealt with. This often involves extending your incision, adding a second suction device, adjusting your retractor, or even obtaining a new retractor (i.e., fixed). *DO WHAT YOU NEED TO IN ORDER TO MAXIMIZE EXPOSURE.*

Take responsibility for the conduct and outcome of the surgery. Some operations are more difficult than others; in almost all cases, good hemostasis is achievable. Blaming the preoperative ASA or NSAID (or chronic renal failure, dialysis, platelet counts that are not perfectly normal, etc.) for bleeding during the operation does not instill confidence in the team. Surgical bleeding should be stopped by the surgeon. Most "medical" bleeding can also be stopped by the surgeon with the appropriate use of the Bovie. *ACT LIKE A SURGEON – TAKE RESPONSIBILITY FOR HEMOSTASIS.*

Almost any bleeding can be temporarily controlled with direct pressure. The use of direct pressure to control hemorrhage while the surgeon gets an extra set of hands, gets better exposure, gets proximal control, gets the proper equipment, etc. is a simple but critical maneuver that all surgeons should have mastered. Do not underestimate simple surgical maneuvers; all surgeons should be facile with them. *THE APPLICATION OF DIRECT PRESSURE CAN TEMPORARILY STOP ALL BLEEDING – REMEMBER THIS, AND TAKE A DEEP BREATH.*

It's amazing how often experienced surgeons can fail to recognize very basic principles that should be intuitive. Blood is affected by gravity. The blood will pool in the most dependent areas; this blood often originates from a much higher point (e.g., the cut surface of the liver with pooling at the base). When called to help another surgeon, one often finds the team working in the area where the blood has pooled, and they are actively missing the site of actual hemorrhage itself (e.g., lap choly bleeding running down the cystic plate, the surgeon cauterizing at the base in the pool of blood). Deal with this in a systematic methodical way. Start at the "top" and slowly work your way down to the dependent areas, controlling as you go. Once you reach the bottom, there will be no more bleeding and no more pool of blood. *BLOOD RUNS DOWNHILL, START AT THE TOP, AND ACHIEVE HEMOSTASIS FROM THE TOP DOWN.*

To stop bleeding you must know where it is coming from. This requires observation of the bleeding. This is intuitive but rarely performed by the team struggling with blood loss. You must get yourself under control first, and then calmly allow the bleeding to occur – observe where it is coming from. This is a skill many surgeons have not mastered because the immediate response is to put a sponge on it, apply pressure, get agitated, remove the sponge quickly, and place a poorly located suture that fails to control the bleeding or makes it worse. Focus this increased energy toward the problem. Stay calm. Remove the sponge and carefully observe. Often a pair of atraumatic pickups can be used to gently grab the tissue where the bleeding is originating from and stop the bleeding, allowing placement of a suture in just the right location. *CALMLY OBSERVE THE BLEEDING SO THAT YOU KNOW WHERE IT IS COMING FROM.*

Do not accept unnecessary bleeding. Even trivial bleeding can add up and become significant in a complex multistage operation. Excess blood interferes with good visualization of the operative field and the identification of tissue planes. One needs to be an expert in electrocautery/Bovie use during surgery. Use of the Bovie should make it possible to stop all unnecessary small volume bleeding. This is often a change in mind-set for some; surgeons must consciously *not* accept blood loss. *DEAL WITH ALL BLEEDING AS IT OCCURS – THIS REQUIRES A CHANGE IN MIND-SET FOR SOME – SMALL BLEEDING BECOMES BIG BLEEDING NOT INFREQUENTLY.*

When, for whatever reason, you are unable to deal with the bleeding with the current team, call for help. Develop a relationship with one or two trusted colleagues that can be relied upon to provide expert assistance when needed. If the situation is poorly controlled and you are struggling, do not hesitate; call for help. Leave your ego at the door when you enter the OR; it's all about the patient and should have nothing to do with your ego or sensitivities. This cannot be overemphasized. *WHEN IN TROUBLE CALL FOR HELP EARLY (BEFORE IT IS TOO LATE).*

If you struggle with certain scenarios or types of bleeding, take remedial action. This requires brutal honesty with yourself. You are a surgeon; the expectation is that you are a master of hemostasis. Your patients all assume this to be the case. Your anesthesiologist assumes this to be the case. Your nursing team assumes this to be the case. Your trainees assume this to be the case. If it is not, you need to identify where the weakness lies and obtain further training. We would all benefit from more CME, especially as it relates to operative technique. *SURGERY IS A COMBINATION OF SCIENCE, PERFORMANCE ART, AND ATHLETICS – IT REQUIRES EXTENSIVE REPITITION AND THOUSANDS OF OPERATING HOURS TO BECOME A TRUE MASTER. IT IS A LIFELONG PURSUIT; IDENTIFY AREAS FOR IMPROVEMENT, AND OBTAIN FURTHUR TRAINING TO MEET ANY GAPS YOU HAVE.*

Take-Home Points
1. Stay calm; you are a surgeon – act like one.
2. Visualize all potential pitfalls in advance like a professional athlete.
3. Maximize exposure when needed.
4. Direct pressure can temporarily stop all bleeding.
5. Take responsibility for surgical hemostasis.
6. Blood runs downhill; act accordingly.

7. Calmly observe where the bleeding originates.
8. Do not accept unnecessary bleeding.
9. Surgery involves lifelong learning; watch masters to improve your skill set.

The surgeon never suffers greater anxiety than when he is called upon to suppress a violent haemorrhage; on no occasion is the reputation of his art so much at stake. J.F.D. Jones

Chapter 3
Endovascular Management of Hemorrhage: Playing Video Games

Jason K. Wong

Case Scenario

An intoxicated 37-year-old male has fallen four stories off of a roof and has a large contrast arterial blush in his spleen and left kidney on imaging. He also displays significant hemorrhagic blushes within his pelvis. He is a "responder" but clearly critically ill…

As much as trauma surgeons love to operate and "cut to cure," they know that not all patients will require surgery. Nonoperative management of patients with severe injuries now plays a critical role. More specifically, minimally invasive endovascular treatments have become the standard of care in many scenarios. These procedures are often performed by "catheter jockeys" (i.e., interventional radiologists (IRs)) and less commonly by other endovascular specialists. Currently, there is limited training in endovascular treatment of hemorrhage within either general surgery or acute care surgery/trauma training programs. As a result, especially in high volume trauma centers, IR is an integral part of the modern trauma team. I often liken endovascular procedures to playing video games, except we get to save lives! Endovascular management requires precise and dexterous hands, while all the information is projected on a screen via real-time x-ray or fluoroscopy (hence the playing video games analogy). This chapter will focus on the endovascular (nonsurgical) management of hemorrhage.

Figure 3.1 demonstrates a conventional angiography unit. Many of these can now be found in a combined fashion with a surgical suite allowing the luxury of the patient to be operated on or have an endovascular procedure all in the same room.

J.K. Wong (✉)

Division of Interventional Radiology, Department of Diagnostic Imaging, Foothills Medical Centre, Calgary, AB, Canada

e-mail: wongjk@ucalgary.ca

© Springer International Publishing AG 2018

C.G. Ball, E. Dixon (eds.), *Treatment of Ongoing Hemorrhage*,

DOI 10.1007/978-3-319-63495-1_3

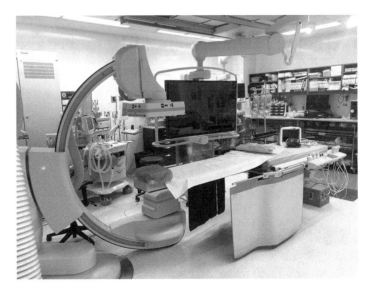

Fig. 3.1 Typical interventional/angiography suite. These can now be seen in a combined fashion in the operating room, allowing conventional open operations or interventional procedures

Role of Radiology

Traditionally, the role of radiology has been primarily focused on diagnosis. Paramount to vital patient care following acute traumatic injury is early diagnosis of the extent and degree of pathology. If a patient presents with significant trauma but is hemodynamically stable, then further evaluation with computed tomography (CT) is indicated. Technological advances with CT imaging have resulted in better spatial and temporal resolution allowing efficient scanning from head to toe within a few seconds. This allows quick diagnoses and subsequent appropriate management in these acutely ill patients with potential life-threatening injuries. In the setting of arterial vascular injury, CT angiography (CTA) is an excellent initial imaging evaluation to detect and define the extent of pathology.

Endovascular Therapy

Through a tiny skin incision and a puncture into a blood vessel, gaining access to the circulation allows manipulation of catheters and other devices to control and stop hemorrhage or exclude vascular injury/pathology from the circulation. One notable example is in the setting of blunt traumatic aortic injury which can be treated

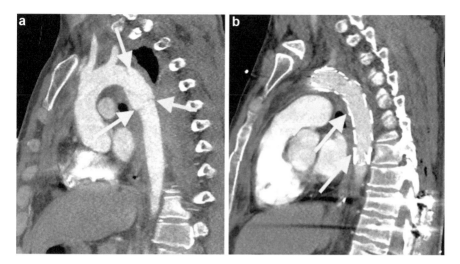

Fig. 3.2 46-year-old man involved in a high-speed MVC with a typical blunt thoracic aortic injury distal to the left subclavian artery ostium (*yellow arrows*) (**a**). Post-stent graft deployment CT image demonstrating exclusion of the BTAI (*yellow arrows*) (**b**)

with an aortic stent graft (Fig. 3.2). So, the question would be "would you rather have a sternotomy or a hole the size of your ring finger in your groin to fix an aortic injury?"

The mainstay of endovascular intervention in acute traumatic patients is exclusion of the arterial injury and/or bleeding from the circulation. Five types of vascular injury can be seen based on imaging appearance: (1) intimal/medial damage with or without associated narrowing of the vessel lumen and creation of a dissection plane, (2) aneurysmal dilation/pseudoaneurysm formation, (3) complete vascular occlusion, (4) arteriovenous (AV) fistula, and (5) complete vascular transection.

Embolic Agents

Depending on the pathology and location, treatment options are tailored to optimally manage the type of arterial injury. Today, there is a vast array of embolic agents available on the market allowing for optimal treatment. In patients with ongoing active hemorrhage, blockage of the bleeding artery just proximal to the site of hemorrhage is one of the most effective ways in achieving hemostasis. It is also important to be quick and efficient. Agents employed to perform this type of procedure include both temporary and permanent products. Gelfoam is the most common temporary agent. This can be made into a Gelfoam slurry where small pieces are cut and mixed with contrast. The ratio of Gelfoam to contrast can be tailored to be

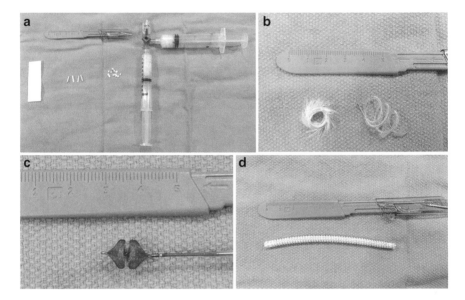

Fig. 3.3 Examples of IR tools. Gelfoam in various states, sheet, torpedoes, cubes, and slurry (mixed with contrast) from left to right (**a**). Two different types of embolization coils (**b**). Note the fibers on the coils to promote blood clotting. Amplatzer vascular plug (**c**). Stent graft, allows preservation of in-line blood flow while excluding injury/bleeding from the circulation (**d**)

delivered to the site of injury accounting for the size of the vessel and how fast the flow is. Larger vessels with higher flow require a more viscous slurry. Alternatively, small Gelfoam "torpedoes" can be cut and delivered. Autologous blood can also be employed where blood is removed from the patient, allowed to clot on the table, and then reintroduced to the site of bleeding. This is rarely used today as it takes time for the blood to clot, and the risk that the clot will dissolve shortly after the procedure is completed is present, resulting in recurrent bleeding. Permanent agents include coils, glue, onyx, vascular plugs, and stent grafts. The IR armamentarium for embolization is large, and each embolic agent has advantages and disadvantages; thus, knowledge of the embolic agent and the site of vascular injury is paramount in choosing the most appropriate agent (Fig. 3.3).

Endovascular Therapy

In the setting of acute trauma, the mainstay of endovascular intervention is to exclude the arterial injury from the circulation (i.e., plug the hole!). There are several ways of using endovascular treatment options to achieve this outcome. Essentially, optimal treatment is tailored to the organ, anatomy, and site/type of injury. One of the most challenging decisions is to choose the appropriate embolic material or device for this specific situation and patient. There may be very subtle nuances in the anatomy that also may alter the decision in choosing between a stent graft and coils and/or other agents.

In patients with partial or complete arterial transection and ongoing hemorrhage, time is of the essence, and stopping the active arterial bleed in a quick fashion is imperative. Hearing clinicians state that "we have finally caught up with the fluid loss" is quietly satisfying when one understands the reality that the endovascular procedure had stopped the bleeding and allowed the "catch up" to occur. The timing of this observation is particularly interesting, as the improvement in patient hemo-dynamics can be quite sudden and dramatic (i.e., only seconds after hemostasis if achieved). For end-organ arterial vessels, selective embolization of the injured or bleeding vessel allows arrest of the ongoing hemorrhage while preserving as much tissue as possible. This allows minimal damage to the organ and thus maximizes function. For example, in the case of a renal injury with active extravasation and bleeding, selective embolization minimizes collateral damage and preserves as many normal functioning nephrons as possible (Fig. 3.4).

Post-traumatic arterial pseudoaneurysms result after disruption to one or two layers of the vessel wall (intima, media, and adventitia). This results in a subsequent higher risk of spontaneous rupture due to the weakened arterial wall. Spontaneous rupture results in a "big bleed," which nobody wants, especially the patient. Thus, early repair/exclusion of the pseudoaneurysm is generally recommended to prevent high morbidity and mortality. Placing a covered endovascular stent across the origin of the pseudoaneurysm is an elegant way of excluding the pseudoaneurysm from the circulation. The benefit of this technique is preservation of the normal circula-tion allowing blood flow to still reach the intended destination. Alternatively, the pseudoaneurysm can be treated by excluding it from the circulation via a permanent embolic agent. This requires "front door and backdoor embolization," where a cath-eter is advanced across the pseudoaneurysm and a distal "backdoor" embolization is completed followed by proximal "front door" embolization (Fig. 3.5). This is an important concept as failure to close the back door may result in filling of the pseu-doaneurysm via collaterals once the proximal portion of the artery is embolized (i.e., the hemodynamics significantly change, and blood flows differently once the proximal vessel is closed). If the proximal portion of the pseudoaneurysm is embo-lized first and collaterals allow filling of the pseudoaneurysm, then it may poten-tially rupture, and there would be no endovascular way of treating anymore as the "front door" is closed.

Trauma to an artery and vein can result in an AV fistula (i.e., a direct abnormal communication between an artery and vein). AV fistulas can rupture as high-flow/pressurized arterial blood is abnormally shunted directly to the vein. Additionally, it may result in steal syndrome, distal ischemia, and longer-term sequelae such as heart failure. AV fistulas can therefore be treated by embolizing the artery proximal to the fistulous communication with the vein (i.e., excluding the abnormal commu-nication from the circulation). For this to be possible, the consequences of emboli-zation must be considered. For example, an AV fistula in the superficial femoral

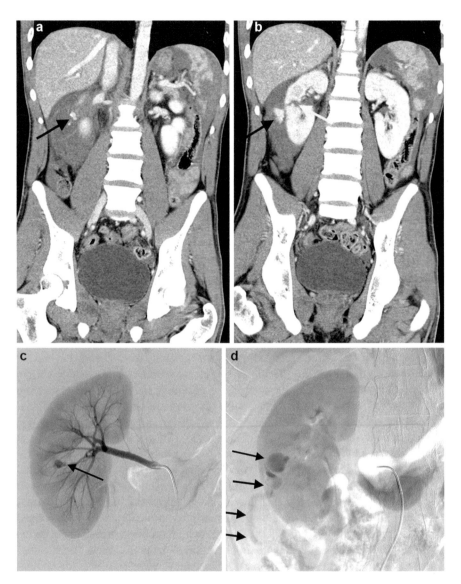

Fig. 3.4 28-year-old man suffering a MVC. CT images demonstrate a right renal injury with active extravasation (*black arrows*). Fracture of the right kidney at the interpole also seen (*yellow arrow*) (**a**, **b**). Angio shows site of injury within the right kidney with active extravasation (*black arrows*) (**c**, **d**). Posttreatment angiography shows deployment of a vascular plug with no further filling of the pseudoaneurysm and bleeding (*black arrow*) (**e**). More delayed angio shows a nephrogram with a small defect in the lower pole kidney in keeping with a small amount of distal infarction (*red arrow*) (**f**)

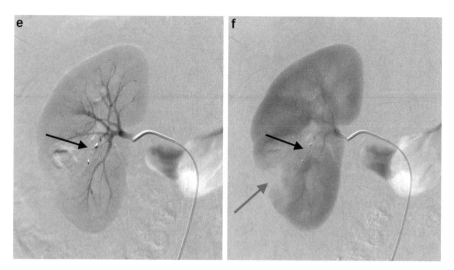

Fig. 3.4 (continued)

artery cannot be treated by this method as there would often be devastating consequences to the lower extremity distal to the site of embolization (as there would be no runoff to the leg). Alternatively placing a covered stent at the abnormal site of communication can also be performed. Consequences of this treatment also need to be considered, as stenting across a joint may cause the stent to deform or fracture secondary to normal range of motion movements causing high stress on the stent.

Trauma can also result in an intimal flap and dissected artery. This can both limit flow and cause downstream ischemia. There may also be weakening of the arterial wall, resulting in potential future aneurysmal dilation and vessel rupture. Negotiating a wire across a dissection flap can be tricky. If this is achieved, then placement of a bare metal stent appropriately treats the injury (Fig. 3.6). In cases of significant injury, where future pseudoaneurysm formation is a consideration, then placement of a covered stent across the lesion is optimal (i.e., improving blood flow through the vessel lumen while reinforcing the arterial wall).

Site-Specific Injuries: Imaging Findings and Interventional Techniques

Head and Neck

Blunt cervical arterial injury has a reported incidence of 10%. Complications include active hemorrhage from an actual traumatic hole in the artery, reduced brain perfusion secondary to vessel narrowing/occlusion, and showering of emboli from

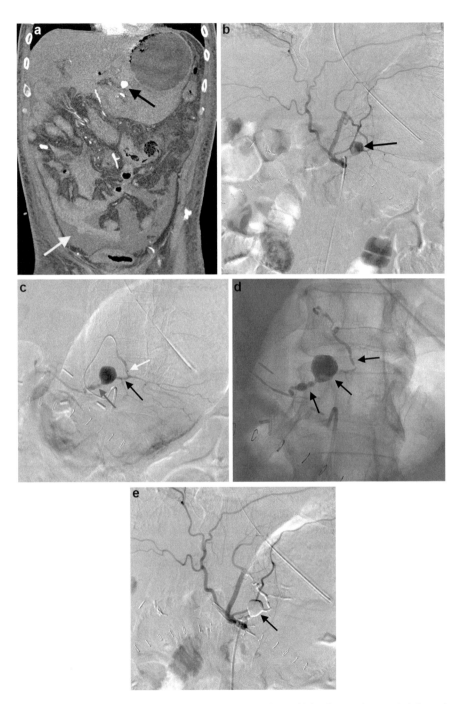

Fig. 3.5 63-year-old postoperative for a Whipple's procedure with inadvertent iatrogenic injury of a branch of the left gastric artery. CT demonstrates a pseudoaneurysm (*black arrow*) and a large hematoma (*red arrows*) (**a**). Selective angiogram of the left gastric artery demonstrates the pseudoaneurysm (*black arrow*) (**b**). Superselective angio shows the pseudoaneurysm being fed by a branch of the left gastric artery "front door" (*black arrow*) and an associated branch distal, "back door" (*red arrow*) and microcatheter parked in the branch just proximal to the pseudoaneurysm

a traumatic pseudoaneurysm or arterial dissection to the brain. Given that the brain is an ultimate end organ (with the heart being the other), early and timely diagnosis is essential to good patient management and outcomes. There is a reported significant associated risk of neurological dysfunction and death (as high as 80%) with these types of injuries. This reality highlights the importance of urgent treatment.

Penetrating trauma results in possible partial or complete arterial transection, pseudoaneurysm formation, vasospasm, and vascular dissection. These types of injuries display the same complication profile as blunt cervical arterial injuries. Significant active arterial extravasation in penetrating injury requires timely intervention to prevent a devastating stroke as the bleeding may be quite brisk. If the internal carotid or vertebral artery is injured, endovascular covered stent placement or open surgical repair is required to maintain blood flow to the brain (Fig. 3.7). If an external carotid artery branch is involved, endovascular treatment can usually be achieved by selective arterial embolization using the agents previously described.

A carotid-cavernous fistula (CCF) may occur in the setting of trauma and is the most common intracranial traumatic fistula. Interestingly, CCFs can be clinically silent for days to weeks following the initial trauma and therefore not recognized at the time of the initial injury. Because the brain is such an important organ, strong consideration for preserving blood flow is mandatory, either arterial stent grafts can be employed or the injury can be tackled from the venous side with embolization.

Ultimately, in the case of arterial neck trauma, preservation of in-line flow to the brain is necessary to prevent a devastating neurological outcome. This excludes the use of endovascular embolic agents that occlude the proximal arterial supply, limiting treatment to stent grafts to treat pseudoaneurysms, active hemorrhage, and transection. In the case of total transection, endovascular treatment requires negotiating a wire across the transection into a distal normal portion of the artery before stent graft placement can be done.

Chest

Blunt thoracic aortic injury (BTAI) is the most worrisome injury within the chest. The mechanism is often sudden high-speed deceleration. In any patient with this suspected injury, emergent evaluation with CTA is highly recommended. The thoracic aorta can be injured at relatively fixed sites. The three shared areas for BTAI is

---

Fig. 3.5 (continued) (*yellow arrow*) (**c**). Embolization of the proximal branch will result in ineffective treatment as the pseudoaneurysm will be perfused from the backdoor branch once the hemodynamics change. Use of glue to exclude the front door, pseudoaneurysm, and back door (*black arrows*) (**d**). Posttreatment angio shows no filling of the pseudoaneurysm (*black arrows*) (**e**)

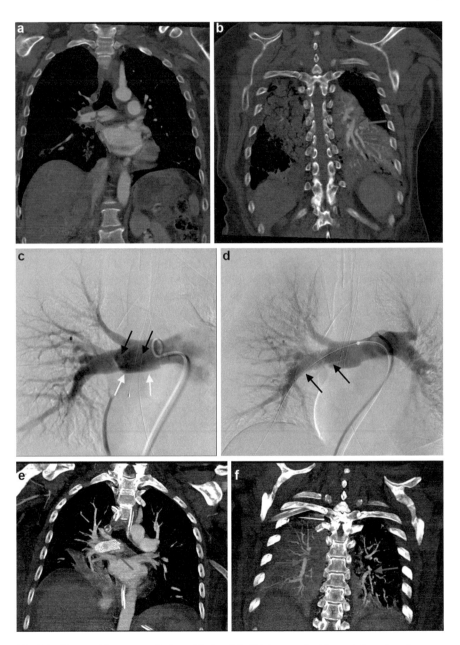

Fig. 3.6 43-year-old woman suffering a 20-foot fall. CT shows a significant right main pulmonary injury with a dissection flap (**a**). CT shows asymmetric perfusion of the lungs with very little filling of the right lung when compared to normal segmental pulmonary arteries on the left (*red arrow*) (**b**). Pulmonary angio shows the dissection flap represented by a linear lucency (*black arrows*) and a pulmonary artery pseudoaneurysm (*yellow arrows*) (**c**). Angio shows placement of stent to tack down the dissection flap (**d**). Posttreatment CT images show the presence of the stent as well as symmetric perfusion of the pulmonary arteries (*red arrows*) (**e, f**)

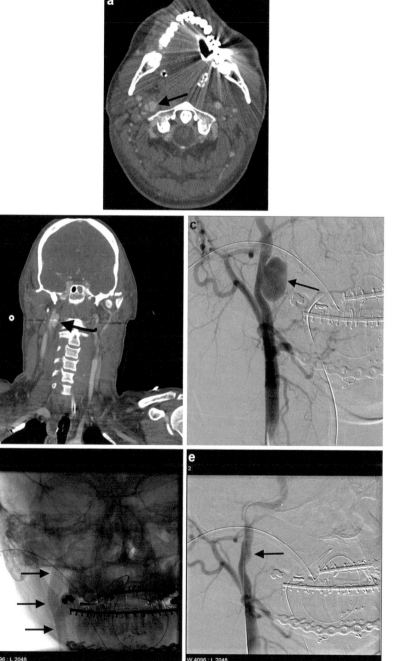

Fig. 3.7 28-year-old man involved in high-speed MVC resulting in a right ICA pseudoaneurysm. Axial CT shows the ICA pseudoaneurysm (**a**), again seen on a coronal image (**b**). Angio nicely demonstrates the anatomy and pseudoaneurysm (*black arrow*) of the right ICA (**c**). Fluoroscopy shows placement of a covered stent graft (*black arrows*) (**d**). Post-stent graft angio shows exclusion of the PSA from the circulation with minimal bulging at the injury site (*black arrow*) (**e**)

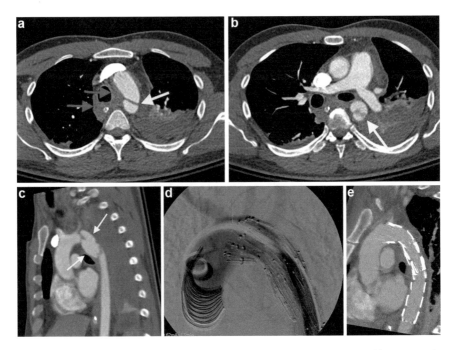

Fig. 3.8 A 38-year-old man involved in a high-speed MVC. CT demonstrates a blunt traumatic aortic injury and pseudoaneurysm formation (*yellow arrows*), associated mediastinal hematoma (*red arrows*), and left pleural effusion (**a–c**). Angio shows deployment of an aortic stent graft with intentional coverage of the left subclavian artery (**d**). Posttreatment CT shows the stent grafts (two overlapping stent grafts are in place) to be in good position (**e**)

at the aortic root, aortic isthmus (just distal to the subclavian artery), and at the thoracoabdominal junction. Patients suffering an aortic root injury most often exsanguinate at the scene of the trauma. Thoracoabdominal aortic injuries are uncommon, and if they occur, patients also often die at the scene. Thus, the most common thoracic aortic injury that presents to the hospital setting is at the aortic isthmus (80–90% of cases) and is located within 2 cm of the left subclavian artery (Fig. 3.8). Commonly described direct signs of aortic injury include the presence of an intimal flap, traumatic pseudoaneurysm, contained rupture, intraluminal mural thrombus, abnormal aortic contour, and sudden change in aortic caliber (aortic "pseudocoarctation"). Indirect findings of acute traumatic injury include periaortic hematoma, mediastinal soft tissue stranding, and hemopericardium.

Patients with BTAI typically require definitive repair. Historically, these patients were treated with open surgery via a sternotomy and placement of an interposition aortic surgical graft. In the last couple of decades, there has been marked and progressive advances in endovascular stent graft technology and treatment techniques facilitating placement of an aortic stent graft for definitive repair of BTAI. Reasonable data now exists for treatment of BTAI with aortic stent grafts when compared to conventional surgical aortic repair. A dominant benefit in this patient population with multiple injuries is that endovascular repair can be performed with minimal invasiveness and with limited administration of heparin which potentially may cause other injured sites to bleed. This returns us to the question, "would you rather have a hole the size of your ring finger for treatment or a full-blown sternotomy for treatment?"

Due to the large size of the thoracic arteries, injuries are highly lethal, requiring timely diagnosis and intervention. Traumatic injury to the great arteries of the aortic arch is most common in the brachiocephalic artery (approximately half of these injuries). The left common carotid and left subclavian are approximately equal in their incidence. Pulmonary vascular (pulmonary artery and vein) and thoracic venous injuries including the superior vena cava are quite rare. Penetrating trauma can also give rise to arteriovenous fistulas (Fig. 3.9).

Abdomen

Intra-abdominal injuries are common with the spleen being the most frequently injured organ in patients with blunt abdominal trauma. CT features of splenic trauma include a laceration/fracture, subcapsular/parenchymal hematoma, and areas of devascularization. Active hemorrhage, pseudoaneurysm, and AV fistula formation are other important findings that can be observed in both splenic injuries and other solid intra-abdominal organs. Traditionally, treatment of significant blunt splenic trauma was splenectomy. However, there is now more emphasis on splenic salvage through nonoperative means given that the spleen has a significant role in immune function. Thus, endovascular management has a key role in the nonoperative management of splenic injuries. The most common technique is embolization of the splenic artery. The splenic artery can be embolized proximally ultimately decreasing the pressure head to the spleen and buying time for the spleen to heal naturally (Fig. 3.10). Collateral arterial flow from short gastrics and epiploic arteries allow sufficient preserving blood flow to the spleen while maintaining splenic function. Alternatively, some centers prefer distal embolization of an intraparenchymal pseudoaneurysm/injury within the spleen (Fig. 3.11). Selective coil embolization is indicated if there is evidence of active extravasation, pseudoaneurysm formation, or an AV fistula. In some cases, both proximal splenic artery and intraparenchymal splenic (distal) site of injury embolization are employed simultaneously.

The liver is the second most common injured solid abdominal organ in blunt trauma. However, morbidity with a liver injury is greater than with splenic injuries. Liver injuries can also present with delayed vascular complications such as AV fistula and/or pseudoaneurysm formation. AV fistulas can appear as early and intense contrast enhancement of the portal/hepatic vein, whereas pseudoaneurysms appear as rounded focal areas of intense enhancement inseparable from arteries.

Intra-arterial catheter angiography and embolization are indicated when CT demonstrates a hepatic injury with contrast extravasation or if AV fistula/pseudoaneurysm formation is present (Fig. 3.12). Hepatic artery embolization is usually well

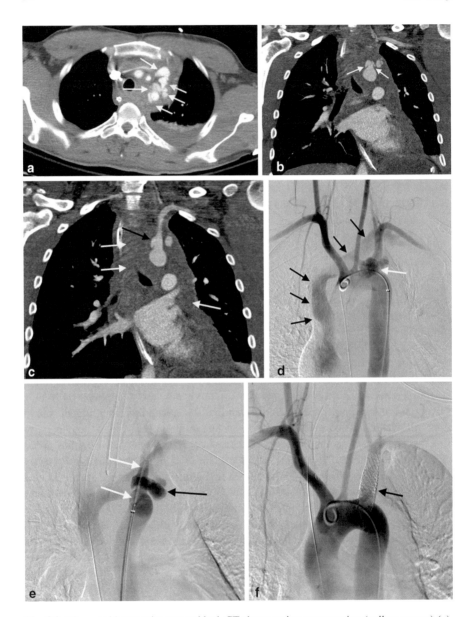

Fig. 3.9 20-year-old man who was stabbed. CT shows active extravasation (*yellow arrows*) (**a**). Associated pseudoaneurysm at origin of the left subclavian artery (*yellow arrows*) and active extravasation (*red arrow*) (**b**). Large mediastinal hematoma seen (*yellow arrows*) and pseudoaneurysm again seen (*black arrow*) (**c**). Angio shows pigtail catheter in the aorta with further characterization of the pseudoaneurysm (*yellow arrow*) and an AV fistula with filling of the left innominate vein and SVC (*black arrows*) (**d**). Undeployed stent graft in good position (*yellow arrows*) across the pseudoaneurysm and active extravasation (*black arrow*) (**e**). Angio shows deployed stent graft with exclusion of the pseudoaneurysm, active extravasation, and AV fistula (veins no longer seen to fill) (*black arrow*) (**f**)

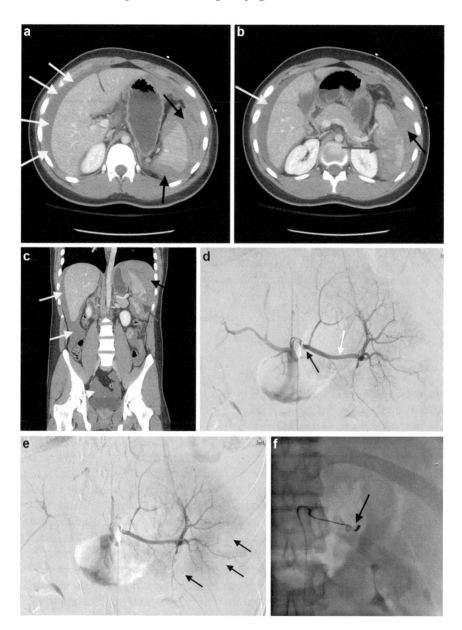

Fig. 3.10 17-year-old man kicked by a horse. Axial and coronal CT images demonstrate a high-grade splenic injury (*red arrows*), perisplenic hematoma (*black arrows*), and hemoperitoneum (*yellow arrows*) (**a–c**). Initial angio shows catheter tip (*black arrow*) in the proximal splenic artery (*white arrow*) (**d**). More delayed angio image shows multiple wedge-shaped lucencies in the spleen consistent with lacerations (*black arrows*) (**e**). Image of coil (*black arrow*) deployment in proximal–mid-splenic artery (**f**). Post-embolization image showing coil pack (*black arrow*) with no filling antegrade from the splenic artery (**g**). Not shown is delayed perfusion of the spleen via short gastrics

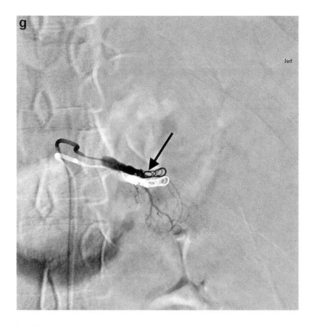

Fig. 3.10 (continued)

tolerated as there is dual blood supply to the liver from both portal vein and hepatic arteries making post-embolization infarction unlikely.

Most traumatic renal injuries consist of small parenchymal contusions and minor superficial lacerations which can be managed conservatively (i.e., don't touch them with surgery or a catheter). However, significant active hemorrhage and renovascular injury can occur and will require more definitive therapy (Fig. 3.4). Distal super-selective arterial embolization may be used to treat hemodynamically unstable patients if there is clinical or CT evidence of ongoing hemorrhage. Stents can be successfully utilized for treatment for main renal artery injuries. If endovascular management of renovascular trauma can be employed, benefits include less invasive means and the preservation of more renal tissue (i.e., nephron-sparing procedure preserving renal function). Significant injuries to a kidney may necessitate proximal renal artery embolization which may equate to an endovascular nephrectomy, as the main renal artery is embolized. Conversely, if there has been significant injury to the main renal artery with dissection and/or thrombus, then time is of the essence to try and restore and reperfuse the kidney with a stent or stent graft.

Endovascular treatment of pancreatic injuries is usually not required. Additionally, traumatic injuries to the abdominal aorta and visceral arteries (celiac, SMA, and IMA) are exceedingly rare (Fig. 3.13). Mesenteric and omental hematomas may occur and are most often self-limiting with nonoperative, non-endovascular, conservative treatment. Iatrogenic injuries can also happen postsurgery and can be treated with endovascular techniques as previously described.

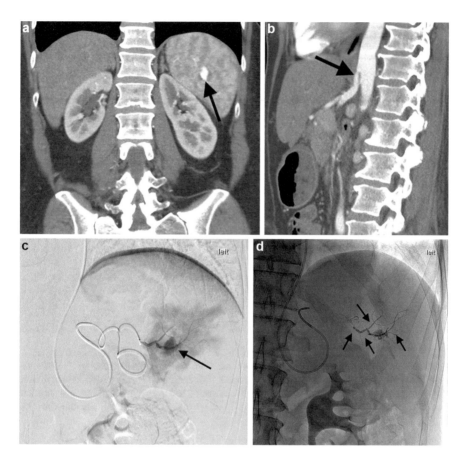

Fig. 3.11 27-year-old woman suffering a skiing splenic injury. Single coronal CT image shows an intrasplenic traumatic pseudoaneurysm (*black arrow*) (**a**). Sagittal CT image shows acute angle (*black arrow*) of the celiac axis making transfemoral access technically difficult to cannulate the celiac axis (**b**). Angio shows transradial approach with superselection of a branch of the splenic artery and visualization of the pseudoaneurysm (*black arrow*) (**c**). Note tortuosity of the splenic artery. Posttreatment image with glue and outlining of splenic branches with glue in them (*black arrows*) and filling of the pseudoaneurysm sac with glue (*red arrow*) (**d**)

Pelvis

The most common life-threatening complication of acute pelvic trauma is arterial bleeding. Although this is most often observed in association with pelvic fractures, isolated arterial injury is possible. Mortality from complications of pelvic fractures can be reduced with closed reduction of the pelvic fractures. Even arterial bleeding will benefit from this maneuver and buy time for more definitive management. Importantly, venous injuries may also show active extravasation on CT and usually

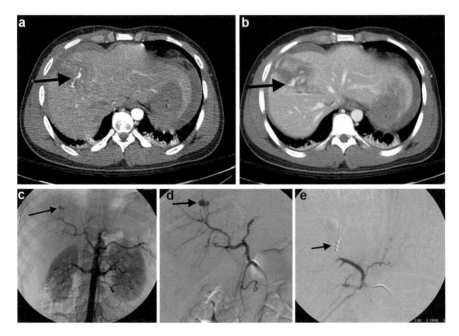

Fig. 3.12 54-year-old woman involved in a MVC. Arterial-phase CT image demonstrates active extravasation (*black arrow*) (**a**). Portal venous-phase CT image shows active change in configuration of the active extravasation (*black arrow*) and a liver laceration (**b**). Pigtail aortic angiogram shows an abnormal ovoid "blush" in the liver (*black arrow*) (**c**). Selective hepatic angiogram again shows the abnormal "blush" and pseudoaneurysm (*black arrow*) (**d**). Posttreatment embolization with microcoils angiogram shows no further filling of the pseudoaneurysm (**e**)

are self-limiting especially if closed reduction with a pelvic binder is successful. If active arterial bleeding is identified on CT scanning, then endovascular treatment is indicated. Shearing forces and fractured bone may disrupt an arterial wall resulting in active bleeding. Superior gluteal, internal pudendal, lateral sacral, iliolumbar, and inferior gluteal arteries are the most common arteries injured in pelvic trauma. Embolization for active hemorrhage following pelvic trauma can be less selective than in other vascular beds, particularly if there is concurrent hemodynamic instability. In fact, some centers perform empiric embolization of both internal iliac arteries if no bleeding site is identified on angiography but there is clinical or preceding CT evidence of active hemorrhage. However, if the patient is hemodynamically stable, then searching for the site of arterial injury or injuries is much preferred as empiric embolization may result in ischemia to pelvic tissue and organs. Correlation with the CT scan is imperative and advancing the catheter to the site of injury with gentle probing and angiography usually will reveal a bleeding site. Arterial injury can present with true dissection, avulsion, and pseudoaneurysms. Often, the injured artery may have a short-segment change in caliber or be truncated (Fig. 3.14). When at all possible, advancing the catheter as distal as possible for embolization is preferred, but again in a hemodynamic unstable patient with

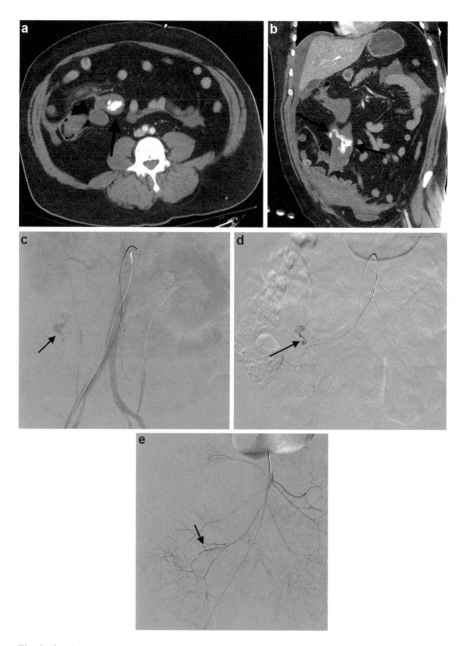

Fig. 3.13 62-year-old man involved in a MVC. Axial and coronal CT images demonstrate active extravasation (*black arrows*) and associated mesenteric hematoma and GI bleed (**a, b**). Selective SMA angiogram shows active extravasation (*black arrow*) from a branch of the ileocolic artery (**c**). Selective ileocolic angiogram again shows active extravasation (**d**). Embolization with microcoils (*black arrow*) of the bleeding branch from the ileocolic artery stops the active extravasation (**e**)

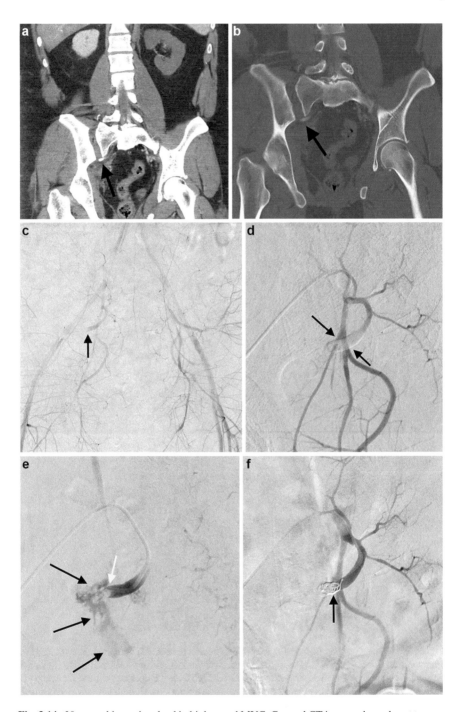

Fig. 3.14 39-year-old man involved in high-speed MVC. Coronal CT images show abrupt truncation of the right superior gluteal artery (**a**, **b**). Also, a left main renal artery injury is present with no enhancement of the left kidney, and there is also marked diastasis of the right SI joint.

evidence of pelvic bleeding and fractures, empiric embolization can be done quickly and efficiently saving the patient's life.

Extremities

The brachial artery is the most commonly injured extremity artery and is classically associated with shoulder/elbow dislocations and humeral fractures. In penetrating trauma, partial or complete arterial disruption can result in active hemorrhage (Fig. 3.15). Blunt trauma usually involves shearing and direct compression forces, resulting in vascular dissection, pseudoaneurysm formation, or even complete transection. AV fistula formation is another potential complication following vascular injury. Again, consideration of downstream consequences is a must. For example, if there is injury to the superficial femoral artery and treatment with a stent graft cannot be completed, then the patient will be much better served with surgery than a proximal embolization (i.e., a potential above-knee amputation). You undeniably lose points for doing something crazy like this!

Summary

Remember to think of your IR colleagues who can play sophisticated "video games" and provide procedures that can control bleeding in a nonoperative manner. Given its minimally invasive catheter-based therapies, IR offers attractive emergency management options for both vascular and solid organ traumas. Even in unstable patients, interventionalists employ rapid, safe, and efficient techniques to control hemorrhage, treat vascular injury, and restore perfusion, which may prove lifesaving. It is for these reasons that including and thinking of endovascular therapy in the setting of trauma early are of utmost importance. Significant delays in triggering endovascular treatment can lead to poor outcomes. In centers with a true hybrid suite (i.e., combined surgical and interventional radiology), we can literally work side by side providing best possible care to this group of sick and injured patients. Sometimes it's even fun!

Fig. 3.14 (continued) Pelvic angiogram confirms the truncated injured right superior gluteal artery (*black arrow*) (**c**). Selective obliquely oriented angiogram of the internal iliac artery again shows the injury (**d**). Marked active extravasation (*black arrows*) with the selective placement and angio of the right superior gluteal artery (*yellow arrow* points to catheter tip) (**e**). Post-coiling (*black arrow*) of the right superior gluteal artery shows successful treatment (**f**)

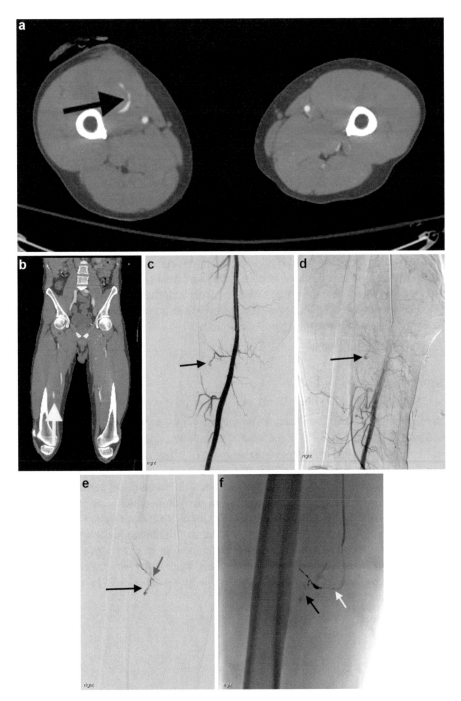

Fig. 3.15 36-year-old who was stabbed in the right thigh. CT shows active extravasation (*black* and *yellow arrows*) and hematoma in the right vastus medialis (**a**, **b**). Selective right SFA angiogram demonstrates active extravasation (*black arrows*) (**c**, **d**). Superselective angiogram with a microcatheter of the bleeding muscular branch off the SFA shows the active extravasation (*black arrow*) and microcatheter tip (*red arrow*) (**e**). Coil embolization pack (*red arrow*) in the muscular branch with the microcatheter pulled back (*yellow arrow*) and near the ostium (*black arrow* shows residual contrast from active extravasation) (**f**)

Take-Home Points

1. Interventional radiology is a key member in the multidisciplinary team approach to trauma patients.
2. IRs are on call 24/7.
3. Endovascular management of significant vascular and solid organ injuries is part of the global approach to hemorrhage.
4. Just like the OR, timely transfer to the angiography suite or hybrid OR/IR suite for unstable patients is hugely beneficial.
5. The most common solid organ to be injured is the spleen. Nonoperative endovascular management of the spleen is a proven technique to deal with hemorrhage and preserve splenic function with a low complication profile.

The aim is to operate only when necessary, but not to delay a necessary operation.
Mosche Schein

Chapter 4
Head and Neck Hemorrhage: What Do I Do Now?

Pradeep Navsaria

Case Scenario

A 17-year-old male has sustained a small-calibre gunshot wound to the left neck. His airway is intact, but a significant volume of blood loss is occurring through the wound itself. He is haemodynamically stable, and you have two other patients involved in the same incident who require operative interventions…

The head and neck are home to numerous essential vital structures, which when injured can ***stop*** any experienced physician or surgeon in his tracks. Securing an airway can be challenging and bleeding can be difficult to control. This 'very little room to manoeuvre' anatomical space when wounded can occlude the airway as a result of direct trauma to the trachea or larynx. Airway occlusion can occur due to an expanding neck haematoma or torrential oropharyngeal bleeding with the added risk of aspiration. Ventilation can be impaired from a tension pneumothorax as the apex of the lungs extends into the base of the neck. The pleural space can easily be breached from a neck wound. Exsanguination from external bleeding is possible from the base of the skull, neck and periclavicular wounds. Exsanguination from internal bleeding is possible from the oropharynx, bleeding into the pleural space, or a massive haemothorax with high-output pleural tube drainage from mediastinal vascular injuries.

It is therefore prudent to establish a definitive airway in patients with actively hemorrhaging facial and neck wounds presenting in shock and a depressed level of consciousness. Oral intubation may be difficult due to airway compression from a large haematoma, bleeding into the naso-, oro- and hypopharynx and direct injury to the laryngotracheal complex resulting in distortion/deviation/obscuration of the

P. Navsaria (✉)
Department of Surgery, Trauma, Groote Schuur Hospital and University of Cape Town, Observatory, Western Cape, South Africa
e-mail: pradeep.navsaria@uct.ac.za

© Springer International Publishing AG 2018
C.G. Ball, E. Dixon (eds.), *Treatment of Ongoing Hemorrhage*,
DOI 10.1007/978-3-319-63495-1_4

45

vocal cords. Surgical cricothyroidotomy is the alternative and should be performed early. Externally bleeding wounds can be temporarily controlled with digital compression and/or a swab on a stick.

Face and Head

Bleeding from facial and scalp lacerations is best managed by early suturing of the wounds.

Scalp

Scalp lacerations may cause torrential bleeding resulting in shock. Bleeding from these wounds can be difficult to control with pressure bandages and is best managed by suturing the first four layers of the *SCALP:* **s**kin, **c**onnective tissue which contains the blood vessels, **a**poneurosis (galea aponeurotica) and **l**oose areolar tissue (contains emissary veins). The **p**eriosteum of the scalp is not included in this mass closure.

Epistaxis

Severe nose bleeds are usually the result of severe blunt midface trauma. The bleeding arises from the depths of the posterior nasal cavity and is caused by the sphenopalatine and ethmoidal vessels. Our stepwise approach is as follows:

1. Ribbon gauze with petroleum jelly or hydroxylated polyvinyl acetate sponge (Merocel®) into each nostril.
2. If bleeding persists, we insert a 10–14 Foley catheter into each nostril into the nasopharynx. The balloon is inflated with 10–15 cc of air or water and pulled tightly against the posterior nose causing tamponade.

Oropharyngeal Bleeding

Once the airway is secured, either by orotracheal intubation or cricothyroidotomy, bleeding from the oropharynx is controlled by packing the oro- and hypopharynx cavity with rolled-up throat or abdominal paediatric swabs. Insert and push these swabs as tightly as possible. A bleeding tongue is best managed by haemostatic suturing of the laceration. Angiography, and embolisation if indicated, is mandatory in patients with bleeding requiring packing of the nose or oropharynx.

Fig. 4.1 Compression of a bleeding vessel/s with a tamponade effect from blown-up Foley catheter balloon

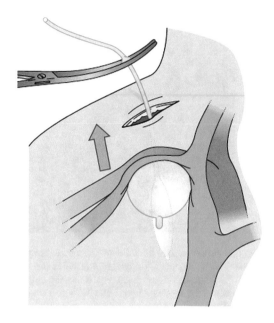

Foley Catheter Balloon Tamponade of Bleeding Neck Wounds

The use of an inflated Foley catheter (FC) balloon to tamponade bleeding is a well-recognised, frequently unutilised technique employed to temporarily arrest bleeding (Fig. 4.1). In a patient presenting with an actively hemorrhaging neck wound, an 18–20-gauge Foley catheter is gently introduced into the bleeding wound, attempting to pass the catheter along the wound tract. No undue force is used to create new tracts and cause any iatrogenic injury. NO attempt is made to cannulate the bleeding vessel; this may occur rarely, purely by chance (Fig. 4.2). The catheter balloon is inflated with 5 mL of water or until resistance is felt. The FC is either clamped or knotted on itself to prevent bleeding through the lumen. The neck wound is sutured around the catheter to secure and prevent expulsion of the FC. More than one FC can be used to arrest the bleeding. Once the patient has haemodynamically stabilised and active hemorrhage has been completely interrupted, a CT angiogram must be performed. Ancillary tests are completed as indicated: patients with arterial injuries confirmed on CT angiography are either subjected to surgery or percutaneous peripheral angiography with embolisation or stenting. Patients with normal CT angiography or confirmed venous injuries are managed in the ward with close monitoring and neck observations.

After 48 h, removal of the FC is attempted in the operating room (Fig. 4.3). Anaesthesia and operating room staff are prepared to proceed to surgery in the event of bleeding. The balloon is deflated, and after 5 min, the catheter is slowly withdrawn. Bleeding at any stage of the procedure warrants induction of general anaesthesia and neck exploration. Figure 4.4 shows the management algorithm for

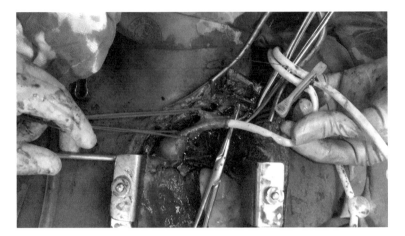

Fig. 4.2 A patient with three Foley catheters to tamponade bleeding from a medial left supracla-vicular incised wound. CT angiogram revealed one of the catheters to be in the brachiocephalic vein, which was confirmed at surgery. It must be emphasised, though, that the rationale for FCBT is to compress a bleeding vessel and NOT to cannulate it, as was inadvertently, albeit luckily, achieved here

patients with penetrating neck injuries in which successful FCBT has been deployed. In the rare event of failure to stop the bleeding with a FC from a neck wound, the patient will require an emergency neck exploration.

Surgical Approaches to a Bleeding Neck

The surgical approach to a bleeding neck wound depends on the area of injury. The anterior triangle of the neck is divided into three zones. These were originally based on patterns of vascular injury.

Zone 1 is the area from the cricoid cartilage to the clavicles. It contains the vessels of the root of the neck: the brachiocephalic trunk, the subclavian arteries, the common carotid arteries, the thyrocervical trunk and the corresponding veins. *Zone 2* is the area from the cricoid cartilage to the angle of the mandible. It contains the common carotid arteries, the internal and external carotid arteries and the internal jugular veins. *Zone 3* is the area from the angle of the mandible to the mastoid process. It contains the distal carotid arteries, the vertebral arteries and the internal jugular veins.

The common-sense surgical approaches are as follows:

1. Zone 1: sternotomy and supraclavicular extension (hockey stick)
2. Zone 2: anterior border sternocleidomastoid muscle
3. Zone 3: anterior border of sternocleidomastoid with mandibulotomy or man-dibular subluxation

However, it must be emphasised that the zone does not correlate well with vis-ceral injury.

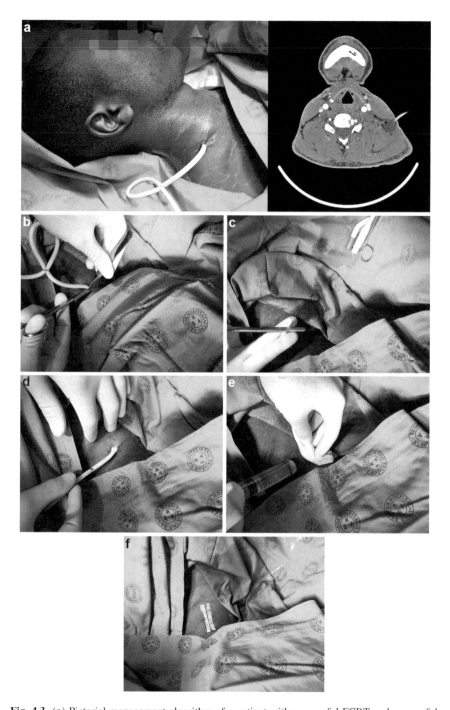

Fig. 4.3 (**a**) Pictorial management algorithm of a patient with successful FCBT and successful 48 h of neck observations. CT angiogram revealed a posterior tract and no vascular injury requiring intervention. After a 48-h observation, patient is taken to the operating room and cleaned and draped awake with anaesthesia and scrub staff waiting in the wings. (**b**) The sutures in the neck wound are removed. (**c**) The Foley bulb is deflated or the catheter is cut to deflate the bulb. (**d**) After 5 min, the catheter is slowly withdrawn. (**e**) The wound is gently irrigated. (**f**) The wound is sutured, closed and dressed

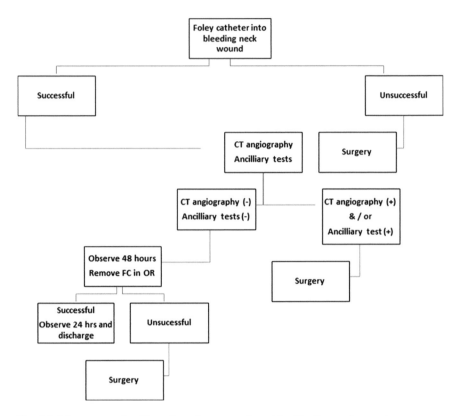

Fig. 4.4 Management algorithm of a patient presenting with a bleeding neck wound

Vertebral Artery Injuries

The extracranial vertebral artery is divided into four regions:

V1: It extends from its origin from the subclavian artery to the foramen of the transverse process of C6.

   These injuries can be ligated or embolised.

V2: The interosseous segment courses within the transverse processes of the cervical vertebrae from C6 to C2.

   Controlling bleeding from this portion can be challenging and extremely difficult. The carotid sheath and visceral contents are retracted medially. The anterior
longitudinal ligament is incised vertically over the vertebral column for the length
of the incision. A periosteal elevator is used to separate the prevertebral fascia, lon-

gus colli and longus capitis muscles away from the vertebral bodies and transverse processes. The vertebral artery lies directly behind the bone forming the anterior border of the canal in the transverse process. This can be removed using a rongeur. Direct ligation is then possible.

OR

A simpler and more practical solution is to plug the hosing vertebral artery with lots of bone wax or lots of haemostatic agents such as Surgicel® or Spongostan™ or lots of gauze swabs, whatever works at the time! This should ideally routinely be followed up with angiography with or without embolisation.

V3: This segment begins at the top of the C2 transverse process and terminates at the base of the skull.

This difficult, almost inaccessible area requires proximal ligation of the artery, packing, prayer and angiography.

V4: This segment extends from the transverse process of C1 to the base of skull and is very difficult to access. It should be managed similar to *V3 segment*.

Angiographic embolisation is the treatment of choice in the majority of patients with vertebral artery injuries as one can see that access can be difficult and time-consuming (Fig. 4.5).

Carotid Artery Injuries

Proximal carotid artery injuries require sternotomy for proximal control.

The facial vein (branch of the internal jugular vein) is the landmark for the carotid bifurcation.

High internal carotid artery injuries are difficult to control when encountered in an emergency neck exploration for bleeding. For maximum exposure of the distal internal carotid artery, the following manoeuvres have been described:

 (i) Extension of the skin incision to the mastoid process, curving posterior to the earlobe.
 (ii) Mandibular subluxation allows an additional 1 cm of working space in the area of the distal internal carotid artery. This is not any easy manoeuvre in the presence of brisk, relentless bleeding from the area. Strong retraction in the upper corner of the wound may be useful.
(iii) Division of the posterior belly of the digastric may be useful.
(iv) Carotid artery ligation, insertion of a Fogarty catheter into the internal carotid artery lumen with inflation of the balloon or even blind insertion of a FC may be the only option to control the bleeding from the carotid artery at the base of the head.

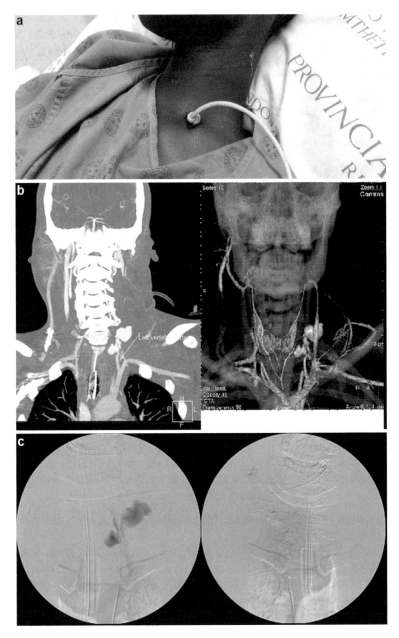

Fig. 4.5 (**a**) Case study: vertebral artery injury. Patient presenting in shock with a stab wound to zone 2 of the neck. Patient stabilises after successful FCBT and fluid resuscitation. Presence of a bruit and FC warranted emergency CTA. (**b**) CTA reveals vertebral artery false aneurysm and arteriovenous fistula. (**c**) Peripheral angiography and embolisation of vertebral artery FA and AVF

Take-Home Points
1. Establish a secure airway early, oral intubation or surgical cricothyroidotomy.
2. Suture scalp wounds and tongue lacerations early to achieve haemostasis.
3. Insert Foley catheter for severe epistaxis.
4. Pack oropharynx and hypopharynx with swabs early.
5. Following digital compression of bleeding neck wounds, insert a FC and inflate balloon; use more than one FC if needed.
6. Perform CTA, peripheral angiography, embolisation and stenting as soon as patient stabilises.

   Two things surgeons fear the most are God and (neck trauma). Henri Mondor

Suggested Reading

1. Mwipatayi BP, Jeffery P, Beningfield SJ, Motale P, Tunnicliffe J, Navsaria PH. Management of extra-cranial vertebral artery injuries. Eur J Vasc Endovasc Surg. 2004;27(2):157–62.
2. Navsaria P, Omoshoro-Jones J, Nicol A. An analysis of 32 surgically managed penetrating carotid artery injuries. Eur J Vasc Endovasc Surg. 2002;24(4):349–55.
3. Navsaria P, Thoma M, Nicol A. Foley catheter balloon tamponade for life-threatening hemorrhage in penetrating neck trauma. World J Surg. 2006 Jul;30(7):1265–8.
4. Thoma M, Navsaria PH, Edu S, Nicol AJ. Analysis of 203 patients with penetrating neck injuries. World J Surg. 2008;32(12):2716–23. doi:10.1007/s00268-008-9766-7.
5. Van Waes OJ, Cheriex KC, Navsaria PH, van Riet PA, Nicol AJ, Vermeulen J. Management of penetrating neck injuries. Br J Surg. 2012;99(Supple 1):149–54. doi:10.1002/bjs.7733.

Chapter 5
Major Pulmonary Hemorrhage: Breathing Underwater

Colin Schieman and Sean C. Grondin

Case Scenario

A 24-year-old male sustains a gunshot wound to the left chest. An initial tube thoracostomy drains 2 L almost immediately. In the operating theater, the hemorrhage is torrential and appears to originate within the pulmonary hilum…

Unique Considerations for Lung Injury and Pulmonary Hemorrhage

Emergency thoracic surgery presents a number of unique diagnostic, physiologic, anesthetic, anatomic, and technical challenges for all surgeons alike. As a result, the trauma surgeon can feel somewhat out of his/her comfort zone when contemplating surgery for major lung injury.

Some of the important challenges common to major lung injuries include (1) patients requiring emergency thoracic surgery are often in dire physiologic distress receiving massive blood product transfusion; (2) hemoptysis is often present in the airways and endotracheal tube causing challenges in ventilation; (3) thoracic operations are rarely performed by the non-thoracic surgeon in an elective setting; (4) patient positioning may be suboptimal; (5) the incisions, instruments, and intrathoracic anatomy may be unfamiliar; (6) exposure will likely be limited by a large inflated lung with air bubbles and blood obscuring the field; (7) associated injuries can be severe; (8) bleeding can be brisk; (9) the inflated lung can be very difficult to handle; and finally (10) the lacerated pulmonary artery is generally not amenable to primary suture repair.

C. Schieman (✉) • S.C. Grondin
Department of Surgery, University of Calgary, Calgary, AB, Canada
e-mail: colin.schieman@ahs.ca

© Springer International Publishing AG 2018
C.G. Ball, E. Dixon (eds.), *Treatment of Ongoing Hemorrhage*,
DOI 10.1007/978-3-319-63495-1_5

There is good news! Most lung injuries require simple technical solutions that you can execute.

Here are the solutions to those problems listed above:

1. Patients requiring emergency thoracic surgery are in major distress. They are in shock. That's why you're here. Resuscitate them aggressively and if needed get them to the operating room quickly.
2. There is often blood in the airways and endotracheal tubes. This is true. A standard endotracheal tube is all that is required. With frequent suctioning (by anesthesia or a colleague), this can generally be managed. If the bleeding into the airways is substantial, you will have to isolate or block the injured side to keep the blood out of the non-injured lung. This will require placement of an endobronchial blocker. You don't have time to worry about this right now, delegate that to anesthesiology or another surgeon and focus on the chest.
3. Thoracic operations are rarely performed by non-thoracic surgeons with who are familiar with the anatomy, instruments, and positioning of the patient. Thankfully in-depth knowledge of the complicated intrapulmonary and mediastinal anatomy that is required for elective surgery is not needed here. Basic instruments, sponges, tissue staplers, and perhaps a large angulated cross clamp will be adequate.
4. Positioning may be suboptimal and exposure in the chest limited by air, blood, and a rigid chest wall. With standard positioning in supine position, a large anterior hemi-clamshell incision, a good assistant, suction, and a sponge stick, you can generally see everything you need to.
5. The inflated lung is difficult to work with, handle, suture, and repair. This is unfortunately one of the greatest challenges to emergent thoracic surgery. In a patient in shock, anesthesiology often utilizes high ventilation pressures, and the compliant lung fills the chest and beyond. Take your time, pack the chest upon entry, assess your injuries, and make a plan. With your assistant squeezing the lung with their hands or a large liver clamp, you can often compress the lung adequately to work on it. Failing that, intermittent apnea from anesthesiology may give you some moments to place some clamps or sutures.
6. The pulmonary artery (PA) is not amenable to primary suture repair. Unlike all other vessels in the body, the PA is extremely thin walled and generally cannot be sutured unless it has been proximally cross-clamped and decompressed, even in ideal elective circumstances. Attempts to suture the wall of the PA when it has blood flow in it will almost always tear and fail and lead to a larger injury. If the central pulmonary arteries are injured most often, the patients have already exsanguinated. If you identify a proximal PA injury, you MUST GET PROXIMAL CONTROL before attempting repair. If this is really the case, you may be forced to perform emergency resection or pneumonectomy

General Principles of Managing Major Bleeding from the Lung

For most readers, the most relevant situation will be major bleeding following trauma. Major bleeding during elective pulmonary surgery has a number of unique considerations, some of which can be generalized, while others remain specific to the pulmonary surgeon.

The general principles are common to most surgical disciplines and will be intuitive to most good surgeons.

1. Anticipation of Trouble Can Save the Patient's Life!

   When the surgeon feels lost in their dissection planes, when tissues are fibrotic and unyielding, when the adrenaline surges, and when your back starts to sweat, those are critical clues that things may be about to go wrong. Unlike in most organ systems, even in highly experienced and skilled hands, pulmonary surgery is defined by the ever-present risk of fatal bleeding. Although it is uncommon, patients can and do die during elective lung operations. This risk is one of the defining features of thoracic surgery and is testament to the highly unforgiving nature of bleeding from the pulmonary artery and the challenges in getting proximal control at the pulmonary hilum. If you feel uncomfortable, extend your incision, let anesthesiology know, have blood in the room, prepare your sutures and clamps, and call a capable assistant.

2. Exposure Is Critical

   The rigid thorax limits exposure and dexterity. Bleeding quickly fills the dependent field, and the risk of further iatrogenic injury to the lung and hilum is significant. When dealing with major bleeding, extend your incision, place one or more rib spreaders, and crank the chest open.

3. Careful Application of Pressure Will Control Virtually All Bleeding from the Lung

   If the surgeon can remain calm and place carefully applied sponge sticks to the hilum or lung, you can almost always get temporary control to take pause and develop a solid plan.

4. Once Temporary Control Is Achieved, Arm Your Battlestations!

   Congratulations! You have stemmed the tide with your sponge, but the fight is just beginning. You must have everything you could ever need at your disposal as you can easily reach a point of no return where repair and success are not possible. Get anesthesia help, blood, sutures, clamps, a second rib spreader, second surgeon, and a second suction.

5. Figure Out How You Can Get Proximal Control

   If you are fortunate, the bleeding will be in the parenchyma or the periphery of the lung. In this scenario, you will be able to place pressure on the bleeding, while a thoracic surgeon or skilled assistant dissects out the hilum and applies a clamp. We prefer an umbilical tape and a Rumel clamp as an atraumatic clamp of the main pulmonary arteries, but large metal right angle vascular clamps will also suffice.

6. Get Distal Vascular Control if You Can

   Often with proximal control, the bleeding will subside sufficiently to assess and either repair or resect the injured lung tissues. If pressure control is working, however, it's good to dissect out and encircle the superior and inferior pulmonary veins and potentially even the distal pulmonary artery. These maneuvers however will be challenging and potentially unsafe for the non-thoracic surgeon, so this step may not be necessary.

7. Assess the Injury and Determine if It Can Be Repaired or if Resection Is Needed

8. Peripheral Injuries Are Simple, So Get On With It!

   Smaller peripheral injuries to the lung are best treated with rapid stapled wedge excision. This is fast, is easy, requires no anatomic dissection, and is often definitive.

9. Central or Hilar Injuries Are DRAMATICALLY More Complicated, Are Often Catastrophic, and May Require Anatomic Dissection of the Pulmonary Artery and Veins Within the Pulmonary Lobes

   This type of dissection is not only challenging under duress, but we believe it is very risky for the non-pulmonary surgeon. As such, for major central injuries unless there is a nice, accessible hole in the pulmonary artery or vein that is amenable to a suture (which is very unlikely), the best management is going to be resection, either with a large "wedge lobectomy" with deeply placed staples or a pneumonectomy. Pneumonectomy in this circumstance involves en masse right angle stapling of the pulmonary hilum, often a crude and imprecise move (Fig. 5.1).

10. Central Vascular Injury During Elective Lung Surgery Can Often Be Controlled Without Need for Pneumonectomy

    In the thoracic surgeon hands, harrowing as this is, familiarity with the anatomy and tissue handling of the pulmonary artery will often allow for precise identification of the injury and suture or stapled control of the segmental PA branches. Rapid dissection of the PA and proximal cross clamp often allow for suture repair of the vessel wall. On the right-hand side, the long length of the right PA allows for more forgiving access to the proximal PA (see Fig. 5.2 below). On the left, the PA is very short, often 1.5 cm or less from the origin to the first branch of the PA, so obtaining proximal control is very difficult. When patients bleed to death during elective lung resection, it is almost always on the left side and almost always from loss of control of a central injury.

11. If You Cannot Get Proximal Control of the Pulmonary Artery, Your Patient Is Likely Going to Die. Your Only Hope Is Emergent Cardiopulmonary Bypass (CPB)

    Once you have lost the option of proximal vascular control, the game is probably up. Most often in managing and recognizing this problem, the patient will have bled to death. If you are fortunate to recognize that you cannot get proximal control, and yet you can still maintain temporary control with pressure, then you need a cardiac surgeon and a bypass machine stat. Emergent placement of the patient on CPB will allow for active recirculation of lost blood and hydrostatic decompression of the heart and pulmonary vessels. The anticoagulation

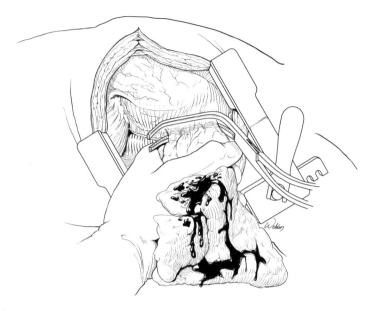

Fig. 5.1 En masse cross-clamping of the entire lung for control of central bleeding (Division of the inferior pulmonary ligament is first required. Left lung in this image) (Reproduced with permission from tfm publishing Ltd. Hirshberg A, Mattox KL. *Top knife: the art & craft of trauma surgery*. Shrewsbury: tfm publishing Ltd.; Ch. 12: p. 177. Copyright © 2005, Asher Hirshberg MD & Kenneth L Mattox MD; Illustrations by Scott Weldon, © 2005, Baylor College of Medicine)

required for CPB is often contraindicated in major trauma. If the cardiac surgeon can obtain major arterial and venous cannulation, then they may have a chance to repair things at the origin of the PA. Unfortunately the requisite combination of temporary control, recognition of a proximal injury, and availability of an emergent cardiovascular surgeon and CPB machine are very rare, and as a result, these are often hopeless injuries.

Making Your Incision and Getting into the Chest

When the decision has been made to proceed to surgery for major chest trauma or bleeding, there is often much uncertainty about exactly what is bleeding, how many organs are bleeding, and how you are going to get exposure to fix things. Further, as listed above, unlike in elective lung surgery, many things are stacked against the surgeon and the patient in the emergency setting. For these reasons, you must call for second surgeon, be it a thoracic surgeon, cardiac surgeon, trauma surgeon, general surgeon, or senior trainee; you will need a skilled pair of second hands for support, exposure, retraction, and assistance.

As a result the trauma surgeon needs an incision that is quick, simple, large, and versatile. This incision is the anterior thoracotomy typically with extension across

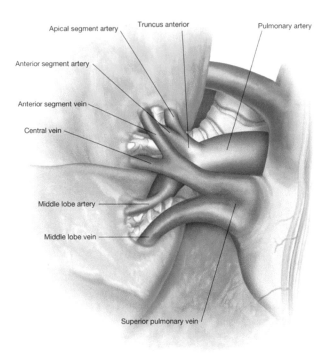

Apical segment artery   Truncus anterior   Pulmonary artery

Anterior segment artery

Anterior segment vein

Central vein

Middle lobe artery

Middle lobe vein

Superior pulmonary vein

Fig. 5.2 Anterior view of the right hilum. Note the relationship of superior pulmonary vein and pulmonary artery (Reproduced with permission. Mathisen D, Morse C. *Master techniques in surgery: thoracic surgery: lung resections, bronchoplasty.* Fischer J. Wolters Kluwer, 2014)

the sternum, the so-called "hemi-clamshell" incision. If the patient is reasonably stable, thoracic surgical help is present, lung isolation is possible, and the injury is clearly isolated to the lung, then a posterolateral thoracotomy in lateral decubitus position is preferred, but often these necessary conditions are not present and may compromise a safe and expedient entry to the thorax.

There is good news. The anterior thoracotomy is fast and easy to perform. The common mistakes include making the incision too small, making it too low, and not extending it across the sternum. The anterior thoracotomy is ideally done with the patient in the standard trauma OR positioning, that is, supine position with arms outstretched and sterile field prepped from the neck to pelvis. Quick placement of a roll beneath the back on the surgical side may provide some additional exposure without complicating things. As a rule, the incision should be higher than you may intuitively think, with the fourth or fifth intercostal space as the desired entry point, roughly corresponding to the nipple or inframammary crease with upward retraction on the breast and soft tissues as you cut in. The incision should be slightly angulated to correspond with the palpable angulation of the ribs, with rapid cuts through the skin, fatty soft tissues, and inferior pectoral fibers and through the intercostal muscles above the rib. Make a large incision, extending to the contralateral edge of

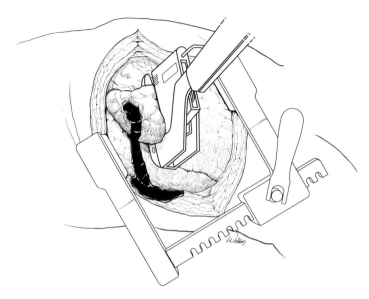

Fig. 5.3 Stapled wedge resection of the lung (Reproduced with permission from tfm publishing Ltd. Hirshberg A, Mattox KL. Top knife: the art & craft of trauma surgery. Shrewsbury: tfm publishing Ltd.; Ch 12: p. 176 Copyright © 2005, Asher Hirshberg MD & Kenneth L Mattox MD; Illustrations by Scott Weldon, © 2005, Baylor College of Medicine)

sternum and posteriorly into the axilla nearing the surgical bed. Once into the chest, rapidly place a rib spreader and begin cranking. The rigidity of the chest wall often limits the exposure here, and almost always the incision should be extended transversely across the sternum with a saw or Lipsky knife. Quickly try and identify and clip or pack the internal mammaries as they will bleed heavily. Placement of two rib spreaders, one on either end of the incision, will greatly enhance exposure with improved spreading and soft tissue retraction. Now you're in, and you're ready to save a life!

Approach to Specific Situations

Major Injury to the Peripheral Lung

As outlined above, injury to the peripheral lung, which for you means the lung tissue you can see and handle, is more forgiving. If the injury is focal, such as that from a penetrating or surgical injury, then rapid placement of mechanical staplers will allow for quick excision (see Fig. 5.3). Alternatively if you have a large raw injured surface or contusion, such as that which may result from a crushing chest wound, rib fractures, major contusion, or shotgun wound, then we would generally advocate for packing of the lung and chest with sponges for 24–48 h to allow resuscitation and clotting. Rarely is resection in this case going to be easy and probably will not be necessary.

Through and Through Gunshot Wound to the Lung

In the rare circumstance of major bleeding from a tubular injury resulting from a gunshot, the often quoted, rarely employed, but clever pulmonary tractotomy may be done to exteriorize and expose the injury (Fig. 5.4a, b). This simple rapid step, utilizing multiple firings of an endomechanical stapler, will open up the large surface area of injury and allow for either selective placement of gentle Prolene sutures or more often pressure packing with sponges to be removed at a later time.

Injury to the Central Lung, Major Pulmonary Vessels, or Hilum

As described above, these unfortunate injuries are often fatal and present a number of technical challenges. Surgery for repair of these injuries completely relies upon rapid proximal control. As described, the mentality and approach will be different when comparing bleeding during elective pulmonary resection and from major penetrating chest trauma. Further, technicalities differ when contrasting left and ride sides. Review of the relevant anatomy is needed. When viewing the hilum from the front, the superior pulmonary veins sit in front of and slightly inferior to the pulmonary artery (Fig. 5.2). The origin of the veins lies slightly lateral to the phrenic nerve. The vein is somewhat flattened front to back, is approximately 2 cm in width, and is robust enough to allow the surgeon to grasp and manipulate the vein to quickly dissect it out with long-handled Metzenbaum scissors. Once encircled, the vein can either be retracted or divided if emergency resection is planned. Beneath and superior to the vein is the large, circular, soft-walled main pulmonary artery. Rapid tearing or cutting of the inferior pulmonary ligament at the base of the lower lobe of the lung is needed to gain access to the hilum and to improve mobility of the entire lung.

On the left the PA is less than 2 cm in length from its origin within the pericardium and the first branch to the upper lobe. To gain additional length, the surgeon should quickly incise the pericardium overlying the hilum centrally to allow intrapericardial dissection and control. Even in expert hands, in non-distress situations, these steps take a few moments and can be challenging.

On the right the PA is much longer, roughly 4 cm, and runs posterior to the superior vena cava before exiting the pericardium. There is often 2–3 cm of PA from the pericardial reflection to the first branch to the upper lobe that can potentially be dissected out without the need to divide and enter the pericardium.

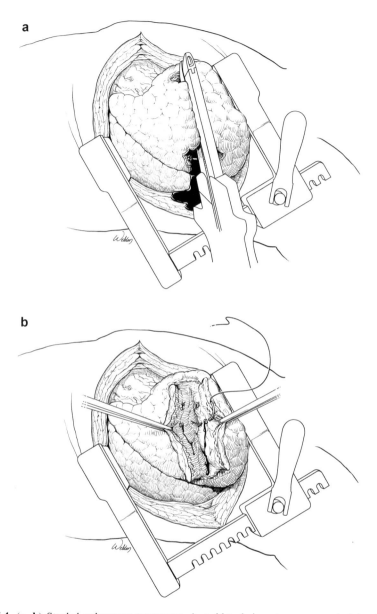

Fig. 5.4 (**a**, **b**) Stapled pulmonary tractotomy. A rapid technique to expose underlying injury (Reproduced with permission from tfm publishing Ltd. Hirshberg A, Mattox KL. Top knife: the art & craft of trauma surgery. Shrewsbury: tfm publishing Ltd.; Ch. 12: p. 175. Copyright © 2005, Asher Hirshberg MD & Kenneth L Mattox MD; Illustrations by Scott Weldon, © 2005, Baylor College of Medicine)

As described above, central/hilar injuries often bleed heavily and are rarely amenable to a simple repair such as suture placement. Emergent proximal control, either with dissection of the pulmonary artery at the hilum or more often proximal/hilar cross-clamping, must be done immediately. Typically this is followed by en mass stapled pneumonectomy (Fig. 5.1).

Special Considerations

Pulmonary Contusion

In the severely injured patient following blunt trauma, the degree of chest wall injury and lung injury can manifest as massive ongoing hemothorax requiring emergent thoracotomy as a stand-alone or often combined operation with trauma laparotomy. In this scenario the lung is often badly contused, as recognizable from the thickened tissue, dark purplish discoloration, weeping of bleed from the surface, and the associated injuries. Unlike in focal injuries from penetrating trauma or iatrogenic surgical injury, pulmonary contusion should not be resected. The contused lung is thick, is fragile, and will not take well to mechanical staplers. Either chest tube drainage alone or if bleeding heavily from the surface pleura, pressure gauze packing of the chest is the most appropriate management.

Role of Thoracoscopy for Major Lung Injury

As has been the thrust in recent decades for acute care surgery and trauma surgery, minimally invasive thoracic surgery has become the most common technique for elective lung surgery. It has however NOT gained acceptance as a useful approach to thoracic trauma for major bleeding because of the lack of visualization from the ventilated lung, lack of tactile feel and manipulation, and difficulty in exposing and manipulating the hilum. Thoracoscopy may be considered for retained hemothoraces, posttraumatic empyema, and thoracoabdominal junctional injuries but not for major lung injury.

Role of Vascular Stenting for Major Bleeding from the Lung

Recent decades have witnessed a dramatic expansion of endovascular techniques for diagnostic and therapeutic interventions for both elective vascular management and emergent vascular bleeding, thrombosis, and aneurysmal rupture. The role of endovascular repair of major bleeding from the lung or hilum has however not gained acceptance as a means of therapy, aside from limited case reports. One can reason that patients with bleeding from the chest rarely have a clearly delineated foci of injury localized to the lung or hilum, often do not have preoperative cross-sectional imaging, often have major associated injuries, and are not well suited to angiographic endovascular stent placement. Further, pulmonary arteries are not as well suited to endovascular stenting given their large caliber, short length, soft walls, and most importantly the need to traverse the heart, tricuspid, and pulmonary valves with the tight angulations and stent equipment. In the current environment, we DO NOT advocate consideration of endovascular stenting for major pulmonary artery injury or major lung injury for cessation of bleeding.

Take-Home Points
1. Most traumatic lung injuries can be managed with chest tube drainage and resuscitation alone.
2. If you're having difficulty ventilating the patient, remember your ABCs. Assess endotracheal tube position and suction out the blood and secretions. Liberally insert a contralateral chest tube for hemothorax or pneumothorax.
3. When it comes to the emergency thoracotomy incision – go big or go home. The anterior hemi-clamshell is fast, simple, and versatile.
4. It's always damage control for major lung injury. Rarely is there a need for delicate complex maneuvers.
5. Call a friend for help.
6. Lung preservation with wedge resections and/or pressure packing is much preferred to large resections.
7. If you can control the bleeding with packing and pressure, that's probably your best move for now.
8. Major hilar injuries are a BIG problem requiring rapid proximal control and cross-clamping of the hilum.
9. Emergency pneumonectomy is generally fatal, but if that's the only solution, then get on with it before the patient bleeds to death.
10. The lung is a forgiving organ. If you can stop the bleeding, the lung will heal in time.

Whenever you encounter massive bleeding, the first thing to remember is that it is not your blood. Raphael Adar

Chapter 6
Cardiac Hemorrhage: Treatment of the Bleeding Heart

Andrew John Nicol

Case Scenario

A 44-year-old male has sustained a single stab wound to the cardiac box. He presents with tamponade physiology, so you open his chest in the emergency department and release the haemopericardium. Your finger is occluding a large anterior cardiac wound...

The heart has been surrounded by an aura of mysticism and romance for centuries. Homer was the first to narrate a cardiac injury in his classic epic, *The Iliad*, around 950 BC. The Greek commander, Idomeneus, killed the Trojan Alkathoos with a spear fixed in his heart that made the end quiver. Claudius Galen (130–200 A.D) recognised the lethality of a perforation to the cardiac ventricles in gladiators, and he noted this to be extremely rapid if the left ventricle was penetrated. Nihilism surrounded these injuries until 1896 when Dr. Ludwig Rehn of Frankfurt successfully sutured a 1.5 cm wound of the right ventricle using finger pressure to control bleeding and a small intestinal needle and silk suture. In 1933 Bigger and Wilkinson described the technique of elevating the superior vena cava with a finger to stop the bleeding and allow the vein to be sutured. Claude Beck from Ohio published a paper in 1943 titled *Further observations on stab wounds of the heart*, describing the best way to stop bleeding from a ventricle is to place a finger upon and not into the wound. These are the surgeons who have courageously laid the foundations for our current techniques in controlling bleeding from the injured heart.

Survival of cardiac bleeding requires clear guidelines on when to intervene, the decision of where to perform the surgery, the adoption of a number of surgical techniques to halt the bleeding, and further resuscitative care in the critical care unit.

A.J. Nicol, MBChB, FCS(SA), PhD (✉)
Department of Surgery, Trauma, Groote Schuur Hospital and University of Cape Town, Observatory, Western Cape, South Africa
e-mail: Andrew.Nicol@uct.ac.za

© Springer International Publishing AG 2018
C.G. Ball, E. Dixon (eds.), *Treatment of Ongoing Hemorrhage*,
DOI 10.1007/978-3-319-63495-1_6

Indications for Emergency Department Thoracotomy (EDT)

1. Hypovolaemic cardiac arrest with signs of life in the preceding 5–10 min
2. Cardiac tamponade
3. Systolic blood pressure <60 mmHg and survival of less than 10 min with major chest hemorrhage
4. Air embolism following penetrating chest wound

Where to Perform the Surgery

The best survival rates for cardiac injuries are achieved in the operating room (OR). Patients have to be sufficiently stable for transfer and be able to survive the period of preparation of operating trays and draping that usually delay surgery in the region of 10–20 min. The OR has the advantage of better lighting and is a far more controlled environment with a scrub nurse providing additional support. What is vital is that the patient should not demise on the way to the operating room as then an EDT should have been performed. Generally the sternal saw is only available in the OR, and as a result exposure to the heart is better. In the majority of trauma centres, the survival rates of EDT vary from 5% to 35%, and the survival rate in the OR should be greater than 90%. The survival rate for stab wounds to the heart is greater than gunshots. Survival in blunt chest trauma is possible (2.5% reported), but patient selection is important with preferable isolated chest trauma and bleeding into the chest drain.

Technique of Emergency Department Thoracotomy

Airway

The patient should be intubated and ventilated.

Anaesthesia

Etomidate 0.3 mg/kg intravenously is the author's preference with morphine 5–10 mg intravenously stat. If the patient moves, then a paralysing agent should be used, but in the majority of cases, an EDT is undertaken in extremis, and there is no movement from the patient.

Thoracotomy Tray

An EDT tray must be sited in the resuscitation area. The essential equipment comprises the following:

Scalpel + blade
Finochietto rib spreader
Toothed forceps
Non-toothed forceps
Mayo scissors
Metzenbaum scissors
Trauma shears (for the clamshell)
Allis clamp (useful for grabbing the pericardial sac)
Satinsky side-biting clamps
Mosquito artery forceps
Needle holder

Surgical Access

The quickest access into the chest is through a left anterolateral thoracotomy in the fifth intercostal space passing just below the nipple in the adult male patient. The skin should be rapidly cleaned.

The medial incision should start at the lateral border of the costal cartilage so as to avoid injury to the internal mammary artery. Such an injury can take a couple of precious minutes to control. The lateral portion of the incision should extend into the mid-axillary line. In the female, the breast must be retracted upwards prior to the skin incision. The pectoralis major muscle is incised. The plan is to get into the chest within 3 min. The incision through the muscle should be in broad strokes, and one should not be too concerned with haemostasis unless there is an obvious muscular bleeder that requires clamping. The intercostal muscles are then identified and incised so that just the parietal pleura remains. A small incision is made into this, and then both thumbs are placed into the chest and the rest of the pleura is opened by spreading the thumbs out in a lateral and medial direction. This avoids unnecessary muscular dissection in the axilla. (Fig. 6.1).

A Finochietto retractor is placed into the wound and the chest is opened. A lung retractor may be required to improve visualisation of the pericardial sac. If this does not improve vision, then the endotracheal tube can be pushed down the right main bronchus to a level of 30 cm at the teeth (Fig. 6.2).

Ensure that the ratchet system is placed laterally so that if there is a need to extend the incision into a clamshell, the retractor is not in the way.

The pericardial sac is elevated in a pair of toothed forceps or an Allis clamp, and a small incision is made into the tented up portion of the pericardium so as to avoid injury to the underlying heart. In the case of a cardiac tamponade, the pericardium

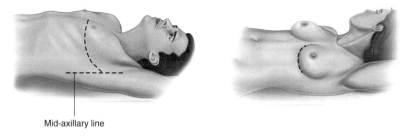

Mid-axillary line

Fig. 6.1 The landmarks for an EDT in the male and female patient

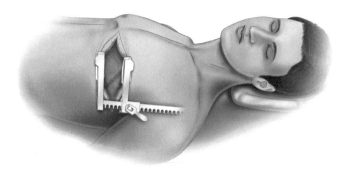

Fig. 6.2 The placement of the Finochietto retractor

may be so tense that it cannot be tented up, in which case a scalpel blade is required to make a small hole in the pericardium. This hole should be done above so as to avoid injury to the phrenic nerve (see Fig. 6.3). The pericardial sac should then be opened up by incising towards the right shoulder of the patient. When the intraperi-cardial portion of the aorta becomes visible, then the incision should be stopped so as to avoid incising into the brachiocephalic vein.

Blood clots should be evacuated into a kidney dish. In the case of active bleeding, the colour of the blood will give an indication as to which side of the heart is injured. The left side will be bright red, while the right side will be a deoxygenised darker hue. Place the digits of your left hand over the surface of the heart in order to stem the flow of the blood. In the majority of cases, the right ventricle is the injured chamber as it forms the majority of the anterior surface of the heart.

In small holes digital pressure is usually effective in staunching the hemorrhage. A finger should be placed onto the wound and not into the hole. If the hole is larger and in the atrium, then a Satinsky clamp may be placed on the hole. This is useful for the right atrium and less so for the left atrium. If this clamp is successful, then place a second clamp slightly below the first and remove the first. This manoeuvre then provides sufficient cardiac tissue for suturing. A Satinsky clamp should not be used on the ventricles as they are too thick walled and the ventricle may be damaged in the process (Fig. 6.4).

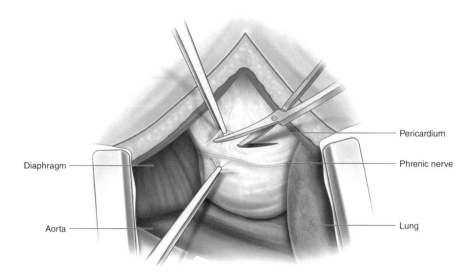

Fig. 6.3 Incision of the pericardial sac above the position of the phrenic nerve

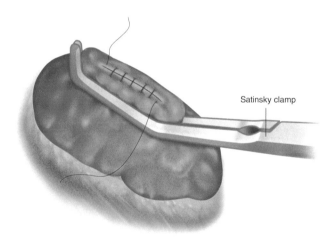

Fig. 6.4 Technique of Satinsky placement on the atrium

Always ensure that you have adequate visualisation of the injury and can identify the positions of the coronary arteries. In wounds entering the right side of the chest and passing through the heart, the access to the cardiac wound may be made easier by performing a right anterolateral thoracotomy through a fifth intercostal incision on the right side. Cutting through the sternum to do a clamshell incision may be needed, and in the clamshell incision, both internal mammary arteries are incised

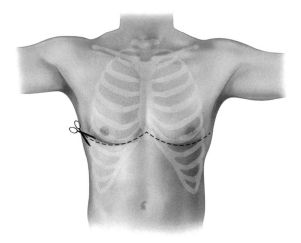

Fig. 6.5 The clamshell

and require ligation. It is important to have adequate access when you are operating, and if you cannot visualise the bleeding source, then a clamshell should be done. In gunshot wounds that transverse the mediastinum and involve both chest cavities, there is often no alternative to a clamshell when doing an EDT (Figs. 6.5 and 6.6).

In large wounds of the heart, a Foley catheter can be inserted and the bulb inflated as a temporary measure to obtain haemostasis. The catheter obviously needs to be clamped with gentle traction. This can be a useful adjunct while awaiting more senior staff to arrive. Sutures can be placed and the Foley removed, and then the sutures are tied.

Technique for Suturing a Cardiac Wound

A single suture should be placed in the middle of the cardiac wound using a 2-0 polypropylene suture on a 26 mm1/2 circle tapered needle. It is important that a large-sized needle is used as the needle needs to pass through onto the other side of the cardiac wound in a single bite. Any attempt to reload the needle usually results in major bleeding and an inability to see. The size of the bite should be at least 3–5 mm on either side. The suture can then be tied, but it is important merely to approximate the cardiac edges and not to strangulate the tissues as the cardiac muscle can tear quite easily and this will then result in an even bigger defect. Teflon pledgets may be used and are placed onto the suture before one places the stitch and again on the needle after passing through the wound. The knot is then secured onto the Teflon pledget. Teflon pledgets should be used on the atria as they are thinner walled but are usually not necessary in the case of the left ventricle.

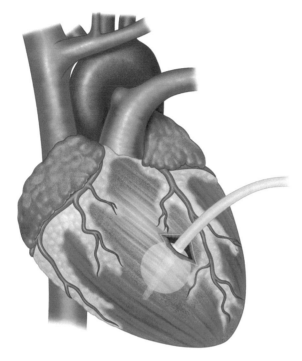

Fig. 6.6 Placement of a Foley catheter into a cardiac wound

Subsequent interrupted sutures are then placed above and below the initial suture as required. Some surgeons prefer not to tie the first suture but to elevate the stitch so as to control hemorrhage and then to place the additional sutures.

A suture may also be placed parallel to the wound on either side and then crossed and tied to control the bleeding (see Fig. 6.7).

Cardiac wounds can also be sutured with horizontal mattress sutures underneath the wound occluding the finger, but care is required to avoid a needlestick injury to the assistant.

Always inspect the posterior wall of the heart to ensure that there is not a through-and-through cardiac injury. When the heart is elevated to inspect the posterior surface, the cardiac output will be reduced significantly, so this manoeuvre cannot be prolonged. A traction suture into the apex of the heart can aid in the visualisation and repair of a posterior wall hole. It may, rarely, be necessary to place the patient on cardiopulmonary bypass for a hole in the posterior atrioventricular groove.

A skin stapler may also be used to control the bleeding from a cardiac wound. The edges of the wound should be compressed and then the wound sutured. This technique has been effective where there is no immediate specialised support. The skin staples should be removed when the patient is taken to theatre and the wound then re-sutured. We do not know the long-term outcome of leaving cardiac wounds stapled (Fig. 6.8).

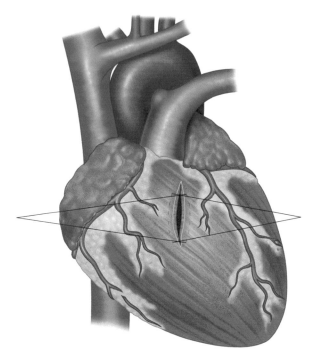

Fig. 6.7 The technique of crossing sutures to gain haemostasis

Technique for Suturing a Wound Adjacent to a Coronary Artery

In this event a mattress suture with pledgets is required. It is important the coronary artery is not caught in the suture. The best way is to start immediately adjacent to the coronary artery and place the first bite directly under vision. After tying the suture, if the heart goes into ventricular fibrillation, then the suture should be cut and the repair attempted again (Fig. 6.9).

Coronary Artery Injuries

Injuries to the distal 1/3 of the left anterior descending artery (LAD) may be ligated. If there is an injury to the LAD in the middle third, then an attempt may be made at ligation. If the heart goes into ventricular fibrillation, then the suture should be cut, and the patient will require an immediate coronary artery bypass. This can be performed on the beating heart or under cardiopulmonary bypass. Injuries to the proximal 1/3 of the LAD are extremely rare as the patient generally does not survive to reach the hospital. If the patient does present, then this injury will require bypass grafting.

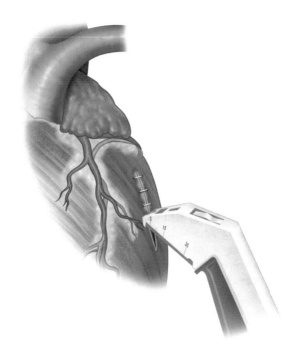

Fig. 6.8 Skin staples applied to a cardiac wound

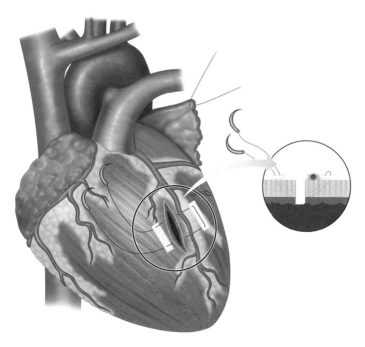

Fig. 6.9 Technique of a horizontal mattress suture repair of a wound adjacent to the left anterior descending coronary artery

Median Sternotomy Versus Anterolateral Thoracotomy

A median sternotomy will provide better exposure to the mediastinal structures comprising the heart, brachiocephalic vein, superior vena cava, common carotid artery and subclavian artery. The only issue is that it will take longer to get access into the chest when compared to an anterolateral thoracotomy. In trauma, exposure is the key to successful surgery and there is no issue if you have done an anterolateral thoracotmy but require better exposure and you then add a median sternotomy. The median sternotomy is an operation that should be done in the operating room.

An anterolateral thoracotomy will provide better exposure to the lung, azygos, and thoracic aorta. As a general rule, if the injury is located between the nipples, then a median sternotomy is more likely to provide better exposure. If the injury is located lateral to the nipple, then an anterolateral thoracotomy is more likely to provide better exposure.

Median Sternotomy in the Operating Theatre

It is important that when the patient reaches the operating room, the surgeon is ready to operate as quickly as possible. The surgeon and the anaesthetist should be gloved and gowned before the anaesthetist begins to administer the general anaesthetic. The reason for this is that many patients will have a cardiorespiratory arrest on induction, and this is particularly evident in patients with cardiac tamponade. The reason for this is that the general anaesthetic causes peripheral vasodilatation, and the positive-pressure ventilation decreases venous return to the heart resulting in decreased filling pressures.

Total Inflow Occlusion

The superior and intrapericardial part of the inferior vena cava may be cross clamped when the hemorrhage is so severe that the surgeon is unable to visualise the source. This manoeuvre may allow for identification and control of the injury. This inflow occlusion may be maintained for 2–3 min, but then the heart will stop.

The Sauerbruch grip is a fast technique to get total inflow occlusion by compressing the vena cava at the junction with the right atrium. The third finger is placed posteriorly to the vena cava and the second finger anteriorly and compressed (Fig. 6.10).

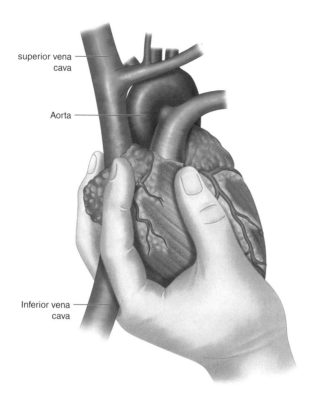

superior vena cava

Aorta

Inferior vena cava

Fig. 6.10 The Sauerbruch grip

Cardiac Arrest and Ventricular Fibrillation

In the event of a cardiac arrest, intracardiac adrenaline 1 mg can be administered directly into the chamber of the right ventricle if there is no venous access. The syringe should be aspirated prior to injection to confirm that the needle is in the chamber. Internal cardiac massage is performed with the left hand is cupped onto the right ventricle to the left of the interventricular groove and the right hand cupped onto the left ventricle to the right of the interventricular groove. The two hands are moved in unison towards each other at a rate of 60 beats per minute. Another option is to place the right hand behind the heart and then to compress the heart against the back of the sternum. A final option is to use a single hand with flat portion of the four fingers on the right ventricle, the cup of the hand under the apex of the heart, and the flat of the thumb placed on the left ventricle. Be careful not to push the point of your finger through the right ventricle (Fig. 6.11).

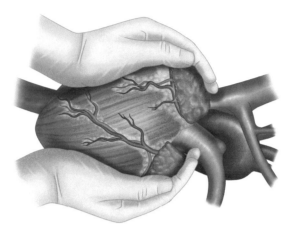

Fig. 6.11 Technique of internal cardiac massage

If the heart goes into fibrillation, then internal paddles should be placed with the one paddle behind and the other in front of the heart, set initially at 10 joules and then increasing to 20.

If the fibrillation persists, then administer amiodarone 150 mg IV by bolus injection. For resistant fibrillation or ventricular tachycardia, amiodarone should be administered in a 5% dextrose infusion of 900 mg over the next 24 h.

Cross Clamping of the Aorta

Cross clamp the aorta if the blood pressure cannot be maintained. The left lung is lifted, and then the operator's hand is passed on the posterior chest wall from lateral to medial. The first tubular structure that is felt is the aorta. Open the parietal pleura overlying the aorta, and place a Satinsky clamp across. This technique is made much easier if a nasogastric tube has been passed to aid in the identification of the oesophagus and avoid any injury (Fig. 6.12).

Intracardiac Defects

In addition to the external cardiac defect, additional intracardiac defects such as traumatic ventricular septal and atrial septal defects, valvular injury with regurgitation, and aortopulmonary fistulas may be present. It is important not to be drawn into long and lengthy repairs. If a thrill is felt, then the acute external injury is dealt with, and echocardiography can be performed at a later stage when the patient's

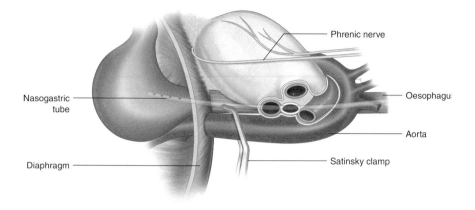

Fig. 6.12 Cross clamping of the aorta through a left anterolateral thoracotomy

coagulopathy has been corrected. The majority of traumatic VSDs and ASDs close spontaneously over a period of 6 weeks, but if they do not, then delayed surgery may be required.

Retained Bullets

Retained pellets and bullet fragments are remarkably well tolerated, and surgical removal should be individualised as to the risk of the removal versus the risk of complication (endocarditis or bullet embolization). One should not be drawn into long complicated procedures in the emergency setting when the patient is haemodynamically unstable.

Conclusion

The prehospital mortality rate of cardiac injuries is in the region of 86%. This means that potential survivors are the ones reaching the ER. It is important that we use our skills in order to save these patients and not wait too long before embarking on an EDT if an indication exists.

Frequently the surgeon's adrenaline surpasses that of the patients, and it is really important to be composed and to operate with a purpose and a direction. If you cannot see the injury, then enlarge the incision.

> *The surgeon never suffers greater anxiety than when he is called upon to suppress a violent hemorrhage and on no occasion is the reputation of his art so much at stake. JFD Jones 1811*

Aphorisms and Quotations for the Surgeon.

Edited by Moshe Schein

Gutenberg Press 2003.

Take-Home Points

1. An emergency department thoracotomy is a life-saving procedure.
2. Use digital pressure initially to identify the source of the bleeding.
3. In cardiac tamponade, make sure you are scrubbed and ready to operate prior to induction of the general anaesthetic.
4. As a general rule, a sternotomy provides the best exposure if the injury is medial to the nipple, and a thoracotomy is better if the injury is lateral to the nipple.
5. Enlarge the incision if you cannot see.

There are 4 degrees of intra-operative hemorrhage: 1. "Why did I get involved in this operation?" 2. "Why did I become a surgeon?" 3. Why did I study to become a doctor?" 4. "Why was I born?". Alexander A. Artemiev

Chapter 7
Thoracic Vascular and Great Vessel Hemorrhage: Big Red and Big Blue

Joseph J. DuBose and Kristofer M. Charlton-Ouw

Case Scenario

A 54-year-old female falls from three stories. She presents to your emergency department with intermittent hypotension and an obvious torn aorta on imaging and no other life-threatening injuries. Her physiology becomes increasingly hostile requiring urgent intervention…

Introduction

Thoracic injuries, in general, are common occurrences following both blunt and penetrating traumas. Despite this prevalence, however, the majority of patients presenting with chest trauma will not require thoracic operative intervention. Appropriate utilization of tube thoracostomy and comprehensive inpatient management will prove definitive treatment for the majority of patients with these injuries.

Patients with confirmed vascular thoracic injury are, in contrast, often a different story. Vascular trauma in the thorax, particularly aortic and great vessel injuries, continues to be associated with high mortality. In fact, many patients with these injuries are not likely to survive to reach a facility capable of providing care. Among those who do make it to care, effective treatment mandates rapid, but careful, consideration of treatment dilemmas, thoughtful decision-making, a comprehensive

J.J. DuBose, MD, FACS, FCCM (✉)
Department of Surgery, Uniformed Services University of the Health Sciences,
University of California, Davis, CA, USA
e-mail: jjd3c@yahoo.com

K.M. Charlton-Ouw, MD, FACS
Department of Cardiothoracic and Vascular Surgery, Memorial Hermann Heart & Vascular
Institute at Texas Medical Center, Houston, TX, USA

© Springer International Publishing AG 2018
C.G. Ball, E. Dixon (eds.), *Treatment of Ongoing Hemorrhage*,
DOI 10.1007/978-3-319-63495-1_7

appreciation of anatomic relationships within the thoracic cavity, and prompt operative intervention, when indicated.

Operative treatment, the focus of this chapter, has changed considerably within the last decade or more. For the purpose of this discussion, open and endovascular approaches and concerns will be introduced separately. In reality, however, these approaches can often be complimentary when employed in hybrid treatments. We will discuss this later in this chapter.

Presentation and Initial Evaluation

Any patient with significant blunt chest trauma or penetrating injury around the chest is at risk for potential vascular injury. The patient or prehospital personnel may provide useful history, but this information is often unreliable, exaggerated, or obscured by what military surgeons call "the fog of war."

Initial evaluation should proceed according to the Advanced Trauma Life Support guidelines, and potentially life-threatening conditions are immediately treated. As with any trauma patient, thorax trauma may necessitate intubation for airway control. While these patients require evaluation and imaging for potential neurologic, intra-abdominal, or extremity trauma, the discussion herein will focus largely on the diagnosis and characterization of thoracic vascular injuries. Physical exam, which should be performed both rapidly and thoroughly, has been shown to be reliable and can help contribute to an accurate diagnosis. The presence of distended neck veins, tracheal deviation, subcutaneous emphysema, chest wall instability, absent breath sounds, or muffled heart sounds may all provide crucial information. Likewise, the absence of an upper extremity pulse suggests a proximal arterial injury. Rapid diagnosis of vascular injury is likely paramount to success.

Penetrating thoracic trauma in a hemodynamically unstable patient warrants operative intervention. The decision regarding surgical exposure may be problematic, especially if there is concomitant abdominal injury. Clinical judgment is paramount in this situation. The hemodynamically stable patient may benefit from additional imaging, especially computed tomography (CT) of the chest, which provides more detailed and organ-specific information.

Initial Imaging

As the emphasis of this discussion is operative management of hemorrhage, we will not dwell at length on the importance of imaging following chest trauma. Suffice it to say, plain radiography of the chest remains the most commonly utilized initial radiographic imaging following thoracic trauma. An adequate plain film should make the diagnosis of any large hemothorax or pneumothorax. Since screening chest x-rays are usually performed supine, however, hemothorax can be somewhat

Fig. 7.1 Chest radiograph of a patient with blunt thoracic aortic injury showing a widened mediastinum and obliteration of the aortic knob

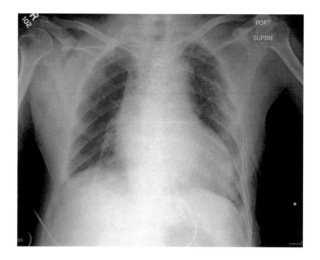

difficult to adequately diagnose. Haziness of one hemithorax, when compared to the other, may be the only real radiographic sign. If this is of any substance, a chest tube should be placed. A chest x-ray may also allow the clinician to evaluate the mediastinum for the possibility of a blunt traumatic aortic injury (BTAI) (Fig. 7.1). A variety of clinical findings may prove suggestive of BTAI, including widened mediastinum, apical capping, or loss of normal radiographic cardiac or aortic arch silhouette. However, none are powerfully specific or sensitive for the presence of BTAI.

CT protocols that utilize angiographic contrast are ubiquitous to initial evaluation protocol of most major trauma centers and have specific benefits with regard to the diagnosis and characterization of vascular injury. While only obtained in the stable patient, this imaging affords both precise evaluation of the aorta and other vascular structures of the chest. The resulting data can prove very useful in operative planning when the situation permits.

Angiography, once considered the "gold standard" for diagnosis of thoracic vascular injuries, has largely been replaced by contrast-enhanced CT. Angiograms are more commonly performed in the operating room at the time of definitive endovascular repair. In this setting, they can prove helpful in defining precisely intraoperative anatomy and guide subsequent endovascular treatment modalities. A key limitation of this modality is the time it takes to muster such capabilities. If thoracic vascular injury is identified in a patient who may be amenable to hybrid or endovascular treatment, it is wise to mobilize the appropriate team for use of angiography early.

Indications for Emergent Operation

The vast majority of traumatic thoracic injuries in stable patients can be managed nonoperatively, but surgery may be indicated emergently, urgently, or in a delayed fashion. Indications for emergent operation thoracic exploration include shock with a penetrating chest injury, initial chest tube output of 1500 cc, or persistent chest tube output of 250 cc per hour over several hours. There is likely a linear relationship between the total amount of thoracic hemorrhage and mortality, necessitating a familiarity of the treating surgeon with the most common exposures that will be required in an emergent setting. The patient's overall clinical condition and astute surgical judgment are of paramount importance when deciding to operate and what type of surgical exposure or approach to utilize. Particularly in the emergent setting, the most important decision is often the choice of incision.

Tip: The Choice of Incision Is a Crucial Decision

Open Surgical Exposure/Incisions

There are several surgical approaches to the thorax, each with key advantages and disadvantages for emergent trauma applications. The surgeon should be familiar will all of them, and the clinical situation should determine the choice of incision. Hemodynamically unstable patients may not tolerate lateral positioning for traditional posterolateral thoracotomy incisions more commonly used for elective thoracic surgery. Compounding the difficulty, the decision for incision may be based upon only a portable chest radiograph, chest tube output, wounding patterns, and mechanism of injury. In emergent scenarios, the surgeon will likely have limited knowledge of potential mediastinal involvement, the projectile's path, or additional cavitary involvement. With penetrating thoracic trauma, there is also the possibility of injury to adjacent body regions, such as the abdomen and neck to consider. Therefore, the chosen initial thoracic incision must prove versatile in accommodating flexibility to provide exposure to rapidly and effectively treat subsequently identified injuries.

In the stable patient, additional imaging in the form of CT may prove very useful. Armed with better understanding of the location and nature of injury, a better decision regarding optimal therapy can be formulated. In the modern endovascular age, this information may also facilitate the effective utilization of less invasive adjuncts, either alone or in support of open surgical means.

Commonly employed open operative approaches include anterolateral thoracotomy, posterolateral thoracotomy, bilateral thoracotomy (or "clamshell thoracotomy"), and median sternotomy (Fig. 7.2). Each approach has its own potential benefits and associated limitations.

The Anterolateral Thoracotomy

The left anterolateral approach—or "the trauma surgeon's handshake with the patient in extremis"—is perhaps the most expedient thoracic incision. It affords immediate control of the distal thoracic aorta and ready control of the proximal left

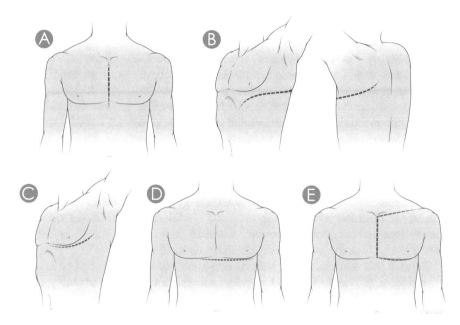

Fig. 7.2 Incisions for thoracic trauma. (**a**) Median sternotomy with right or left neck extensions can be used to treat injuries to the heart, proximal aorta, and innominate and left carotid arteries. (**b**) Left posterolateral thoracotomy for repair of descending thoracic aortic injuries. (**c**) Left anterolateral thoracotomy for patients in extremis (ED thoracotomy) also provides access to the left subclavian artery. (**d**) Extension of the anterolateral thoracotomy to the opposite chest as a "clamshell" incision. (**e**) "Book" thoracotomy

subclavian artery origin at the apex of the thoracic cavity on the left. The heart can also be readily accessed from this incision, allowing evacuation of hemopericardium and effective cardiac compressions—or even direct cardiac repair, in select situations.

External landmarks are the most reliable expedient means of identifying optimal incision orientation. The incision is initiated just below the nipple in males and extends from the lateral aspect of the sternum along the curvature of the rib into the axilla. By extending the ipsilateral arm and placing a bump to elevate the thorax approximately 20°, the incision can be carried optimally posteriorly—a maneuver that will improve posterior exposure. If required, this incision can be extended across the midline into a "clamshell thoracotomy." The main disadvantage of the anterolateral approach is exposure of posterior thoracic structures. The posterolateral thoracotomy allows better exposure of the hemithorax, especially the posterior structures, and is the standard incision for most elective thorax operations. The posterior lateral incision, however, lacks of versatility and has limited usefulness in the emergent setting. It may, however, prove the preferred approach in more stable patients who require exposure and treatment of intrathoracic tracheoesophageal injuries.

Clamshell Thoracotomy

The previously described "clamshell thoracotomy" extension of the anterolateral thoracotomy across the sternum is a maneuver that affords excellent exposure to both pleural spaces, the anterior mediastinum, and nearly the full complement of thoracic vascular structures. The incision is a mirror of the anterior lateral thoracotomy but on the right side. The sternum can be divided using a Lebsche knife or trauma shears to connect the two incisions.

In practice, if no imaging is available to guide incision selection in a patient in extremis, the lead surgeon should instruct another capable member of the team to place a right thoracostomy tube simultaneous to the left anterolateral thoracotomy. If the blood is identified upon right thoracostomy tube placement, then the left anterolateral incision is immediately extended to a "clamshell" incision. Other very experienced authors advocate routine "clamshell" thoracotomy for all patients in extremis who have the potential for significant thoracic injury.

Extension of the "clamshell" incision into a midline laparotomy can be accomplished via a "T" extension onto the abdominal wall. There is limited ability, however, to extend into the neck with this particular incision. As a result, separate neck incisions along the sternocleidomastoid are typically utilized when required.

Median Sternotomy

Median sternotomy is a commonly utilized incision of elective cardiac surgery and is very effective in facilitating excellent access to the heart, proximal great vessels, and anterior mediastinum. This particular incision is also versatile and can be extended as an abdominal, periclavicular, or neck incision. Division of the sternum along its long axis can, however, take more time than the "clamshell" exposure variant of mediastinal exposure.

An additional extension of the median sternotomy includes the "trap door" approach, whereby an anterolateral thoracotomy is combined with a median sternotomy (most commonly on the left) to facilitate improved exposure to the proximal course of thoracic vessels. In practice, this incision is rarely utilized, however, as similar exposure can be obtained with the combination of a median sternotomy and a periclavicular incision.

Periclavicular Incisions (Supraclavicular, Infraclavicular, and Trans-Clavicular)

The clavicle effectively guards the mid-subclavian artery from expedient surgical exposure bilaterally. Exposure of this region may also afford control of the proximal vertebral arteries, should they require it. Options for improved exposure of this area include incisions above, through, or below the clavicle.

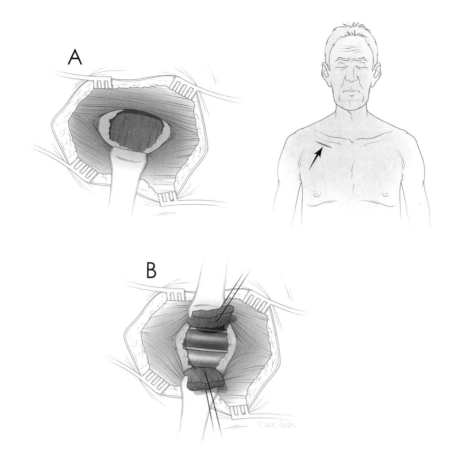

Fig. 7.3 Infra-clavicular exposure of the subclavian artery and vein

Infraclavicular incisions are limited by their ability to afford wide exposure without significant division of the pectoralis major but can prove effective in rapidly facilitating vascular control of junctional hemorrhage of either proximal arm. To facilitate this control, an incision is made approximately one fingerbreadth below the middle of the clavicle. The pectoralis major fibers are identified and splint, exposing the underlying pectoralis minor. This muscle is then encircled and divided, exposing the distal subclavian/proximal axillary artery for clamping and control (Fig. 7.3a, b).

Supraclavicular access of the subclavian artery (Fig. 7.4a, b) can be achieved by making an incision approximately one fingerbreadth above the clavicle, centered on the medial (or clavicular) head of the sternocleidomastoid (SCM) muscle. This medial head of the SCM is then divided, revealing the jugular vein medially and the anterior scalene directly under the medial SCM head. Overlying this muscle, traveling from lateral to medial (unlike most nerves that travel medial to lateral in surgical

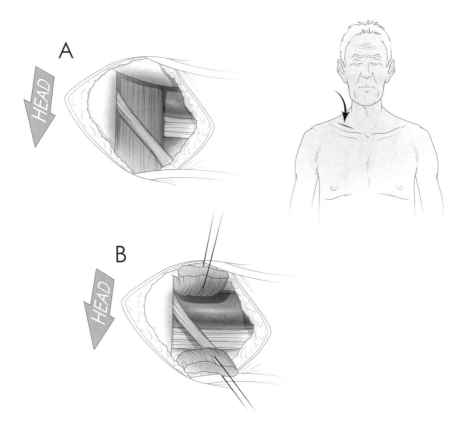

Fig. 7.4 Supraclavicular approach to the subclavian artery. The clavicular head of the sternoclei-domastoid has been divided, exposing the anterior scalene and overlying phrenic nerve; (**a**) with resection of the anterior scalene (the phrenic is preserved and protected), the underlying subclavian artery is exposed (**b**) division of the anterior scalene muscle, revealing the underlying subclavian artery above the clavicle

fields) is the phrenic nerve. This nerve is preserved and the anterior scalene is divided. This reveals the underlying subclavian artery, which can be effectively controlled.

The transclavicular approach perhaps affords the widest and most effective expo-sure of the subclavian artery. This is accomplished by an incision directly over the clavicle. The ligaments of the clavicular head can then be divided using a scalpel or scissors. However, these attachments are notoriously dense and problematic. Obtaining circumferential control of the mid-clavicle and dividing it with a Gigli saw may facilitate a more expedient and effective exposure. Subsequent reflection of the clavicle affords excellent exposure of the subclavian vein and artery as well as the proximal common carotid (particularly on the right side) (Fig. 7.5a, b).

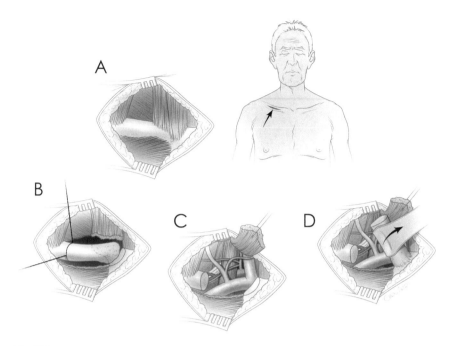

Fig. 7.5 Resection of the clavicle with subsequent exposure of the subclavian artery (**a–c**). As an alternative, the clavicular head can be left in place after clavicle resection, with cranial reflection of the head (**d**)

A Brief Word About Anomalies

Anomalies of the thoracic vasculature are not exceptionally rare. Because they can be encountered in the trauma setting, they are worth mentioning here. The most common is referred to as the "bovine arch," where the left common carotid artery originates from the innominate artery instead of the aortic arch. Next, in order of frequency, is the left vertebral artery, which originates directly from the aortic arch (as opposed to from the proximal subclavian), followed by the replaced right subclavian artery, originating from the thoracic aorta distal to the left subclavian. In the majority of instances, these will be of little consequence to the issue at hand during significant vascular trauma. The one important situation that may occur is when endovascular stent graft coverage of a thoracic aortic injury is being considered in the setting of a replaced right subclavian. In this setting, coverage of the aortic injury may necessitate coverage of the aberrant vessel and subsequent vascular bypass.

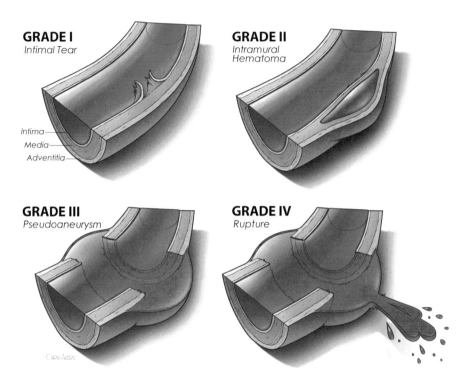

Classification of
TRAUMATIC AORTIC INJURY

Fig. 7.6 Classification of traumatic aortic injury

Management of Specific Thoracic Vascular Injuries

Blunt Thoracic Aortic Injury

BTAI remains the second most frequent cause of mortality, after blunt force, and, in many ways, is the "signature" vascular thoracic injury. Autopsy studies suggest that the majority of patients with severe BTAI will not survive to reach a medical facility. Among those who do, a full spectrum of injury severity may be encountered. BTAIs represent a spectrum of lesions that range from intimal tears to free rupture. The mechanism often involves rapid deceleration, where the greatest point of strain is at the aortic isthmus, explaining the most common site of injury—just distal to the left subclavian artery. Classification of BTAI is based on the extent of injury to the anatomic layers of the aortic wall. Based on imaging, BTAI is classified into four grades: intimal tears (grade 1), intramural hematoma (grade 2), pseudoaneurysm (grade 3), and rupture (grade 4) (Fig. 7.6).

Grade 1 injuries do not cause an external aortic contour abnormality and are best visualized on CTA or intravascular ultrasound. Injuries involving the media, such as intramural hematomas or dissections, are considered grade 2. Pseudoaneurysms and ruptures (grades 3 and 4, respectively) are easily visualized using imaging modalities. While additional classification systems based on contemporary imaging have also been proposed, accurate characterization of BTAI severity is critical because it affects management decisions.

As opposed to many other forms of vascular injury, there is an abundance of data that suggests that endovascular repair is superior to open repair of thoracic aortic injuries. Thoracic endovascular aortic repair (TEVAR) has emerged as the primary treatment modality utilized for TAI among amenable patients. It is important to note, however, that not all BTAIs require repair. Even those that do require operative intervention do not typically undergo TEVAR in the emergent setting.

Immediate management of all BTAI injuries, either as definitive therapy or during preparation for repair, includes aggressive blood pressure control. Effective pharmacologic suppression of aortic pressure fluctuations is utilized to reduce the stress on the injured aortic wall. For grade 1 injuries, medical management alone is the mainstay of definitive therapy. For grades 2, 3, and 4 injuries, current guidelines by the Society for Vascular Surgery suggest medical management be utilized as a bridge to subsequent repair. The optimal blood pressure goal and control regiment have not been well established, but the authors utilize a systolic blood pressure less than 120 mm Hg as a desired goal. We use short-acting beta-blockers that can be titrated to achieve this objective.

It is important to consider that specific patterns of associated traumatic injury may affect the ability to employ medical therapy for BTAI. Specifically, patients with traumatic brain injury requiring optimization of cerebral perfusion pressure (CPP) may require elevation of blood pressure to optimize neurologic outcome. This required elevation is counter to the medical management of BTAI and may necessitate earlier intervention for aortic injury to facilitate optimal brain injury outcome. Given the common complexity of severely injured trauma patients, it is advisable that all discussions about the appropriateness of medical therapy and timing of potential BTAI repair be undertaken in a collaborative fashion by the key stakeholders in care.

BTAI Repair

While prompt repair of BTAI is preferred, existing data suggests that selective delayed repair may result in optimal outcomes. This approach is commonly required among trauma patients requiring treatment of more immediate life-threatening injuries, such as laparotomy or emergent craniotomy—a common occurrence among the severely injured cohort. Until definitive intervention for BTAI is undertaken, medical management of blood pressure control is performed in an appropriate intensive care setting. The subsequent timing of definitive repair is then individualized for the specific patient through a multidisciplinary, decision-making process.

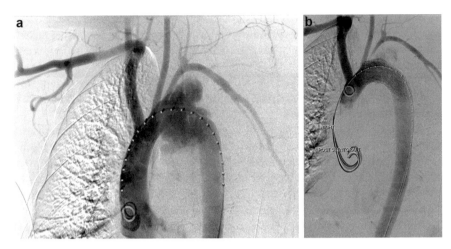

Fig. 7.7 (**a**) Diagnostic and (**b**) completion angiography of a patient with a grade 3 blunt thoracic aortic injury

The technique utilized for endovascular repair is multifaceted. In summary, endovascular repair is usually performed under general anesthesia in a hybrid operating room equipped with fixed imaging equipment. Intraoperatively, the abdomen and bilateral groins are prepped in standard fashion. An arch aortogram is performed through femoral access, and the location of the injury is confirmed. The cerebrovascular anatomy is evaluated based on the arch angiogram, especially if left subclavian artery coverage is planned. The patient is anticoagulated using a weight-based heparin protocol if there are no contraindications. Otherwise, a smaller dose of heparin (3000–5000 units) is administered.

The thoracic device is selected based on CT images according to the manufacturer's sizing recommendations. Measurements are made based on two-dimensional, thin-cut axial CT scans with IV contrast. The device is delivered and deployed, and extension pieces are utilized as indicated to cover the area of injury. The subclavian artery is covered, as needed, to obtain a proximal landing zone or gain better apposition with the lesser curvature of the aortic arch. We maintain a policy of selective delayed subclavian artery revascularization for such cases, as the majority of trauma patients tolerate left subclavian coverage without adverse event. Post-deployment balloon angioplasty is performed selectively when incomplete apposition of the graft at the proximal landing zone is noted (Fig. 7.7a, b). The heparin is then reversed with protamine. Postoperatively, patients are returned to the surgical-trauma intensive care unit and discharged following stabilization of their other injuries.

Even though endovascular repair has largely supplanted open approaches for BTAI treatment, select patients with unsuitable anatomy or other confounding factors may continue to require open surgical intervention. In the modern era, open surgery is reserved for specific scenarios. Among patients showing signs of hemodynamic compromise and the need for emergent repair, not all facilities will have the capability to martial endovascular resources in the required time frame to optimize outcome. While rapid mobilization of endovascular resources is inherent to many modern trauma centers, local capabilities must be considered—and may be a limitation to endovascular utilization when required emergently.

Other considerations in selecting open repair include the consideration of patients anatomically unfavorable for TEVAR. The foremost criterion determining the need for open repair is the absence of an adequate proximal landing zone to allow for proper "seal" of the site of injury by the device. In approximately 40% of BTAI patients, left subclavian artery coverage is required to achieve this objective. Available data suggests that the majority of trauma patients requiring left subclavian artery coverage in this setting will have good short- and mid-term outcomes without the need for subsequent bypass. Other anatomical criteria that may preclude the ability to safely conduct TEVAR for BTAI include small or diseased iliofemoral vessels, as diameter of these vessels of less than 7 mm is a risk factor for access site complications, including dissection, rupture, and hematoma formation.

When open repair is required, a number of approaches can be considered to facilitate BTAI treatment, depending on the site and length of the descending thoracic aorta involved. Given that the most commonly encountered location of BTAI is in the region of the isthmus, a left posterolateral thoracotomy to enter the chest through the fourth space is usually the most expedient—regarded as the optimal incision choice to address this specific injury. Once the chest is opened, the initial objective is to acquire proximal and distal control around the area of injured thoracic aorta. The proximal clamp is typically applied between the left common carotid and left subclavian arteries, while the distal clamp is placed at some point on the distal descending thoracic aorta distal to the zone of injury.

Depending on the clinical scenario and patient condition, a distal aortic perfusion strategy should be expediently developed. The most expeditious technique is "left heart bypass," which can be performed through cannulation of the left inferior pulmonary vein and distal thoracic aorta (Fig. 7.8). Rarely, the proximal clamp positioning is untenable. In this scenario, full cardiopulmonary bypass (CPB) is more ideal, commonly through a femoral artery and a femoral vein cannulation.

One of the caveats, which is often problematic for the polytrauma patient, is the need for systemic anticoagulation with the use of bypass. For left heart bypass, this is achieved through administration of intravenous heparin at a dose of 1 mg/kg to achieve an activated clotting time (ACT) of more than 200 s. In cases where full bypass is required, heparin is used at a dose of 4 mg/Kg to achieve an ACT of greater than 480 s. Once the patient is on bypass and the perfusion circuit is satisfactory, the periaortic hematoma is incised, the extent of injury explored, and the ensuing aortic repair with synthetic graft undertaken. It is paramount that the aortic adventitia is incorporated into the subsequent suture lines, as this layer provides the majority of the tensile strength of the aorta. The patient is gradually rewarmed during the latter phase of the anastomosis to facilitate removal of the clamps at a moderate degree of hypothermia (32–34 °C).

A significant consideration when undertaking open BTAI repair is spinal cord protection and the importance of distal aortic perfusion in minimizing the risk of postoperative paraplegia. Several potential strategies designed to mitigate the risk of

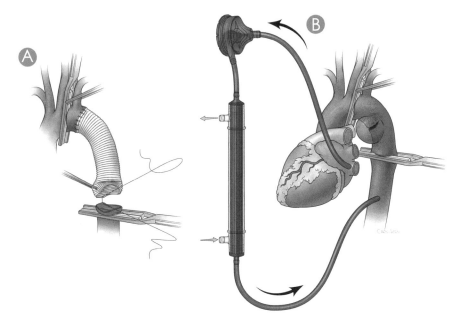

Fig. 7.8 Open repair of blunt thoracic aortic injury can be performed using a (**a**) clamp and sew technique or (**b**) distal aortic perfusion

postoperative paraplegia exist. Perhaps the most significant contributor to spinal cord ischemia occurs as a result of aortic clamping and subsequent occlusion of critical segmental spinal cord arterial branches. Important factors in determining the incidence of immediate onset or delayed paraplegia following aortic repair include duration of cross clamping, level and length of aortic segment excluded by clamping, duration of systemic hypotension, cerebrospinal fluid pressure, distal aortic pressure, and the number of intercostals ligated during repair. Multiple adjuncts have helped lower the incidence of paraplegia following aortic repair for BTAI, including cerebrospinal fluid drainage, administration of steroids, generalized and localized hypothermia, as well as reattachment of key intercostal arteries during the conduct of repair.

Potential Complications of TEVAR

Although TEVAR has proven a superior option to open repair for most BTAI patients, there are important complications of TEVAR to consider. While they occur less commonly than in open surgical repair, stroke and paralysis are devastating (but fortunately rare) potential risks. Vascular access- and device-related complications are also rare, but real, complications of TEVAR in contemporary practice.

Excessive oversizing or undersizing of endografts can lead to propagation of aortic injury or failure to achieve adequate seal. Patient-specific anatomical issues may also contribute, including the presence of a tight curvature of the aortic arch, the native atherosclerotic burden, and the aforementioned diameter limitations of iliac access vessels.

Vascular Injuries to the Aortic Arch Vessels and Thoracic Outlet Vasculature

While TAI is perhaps the hallmark thoracic vascular injury, a wide variety of traumatic pathologies at various vascular structures within the chest can be encountered. The majority of these injuries are initially diagnosed with contrast-enhanced CT, now ubiquitous to initial trauma evaluations. As with BTAI, the patient condition and associated injuries remain considerations in defining optimal management of identified vascular injuries. For unstable patients requiring immediate surgical intervention, particularly after penetrating mechanisms, initial open repair approaches are commonly utilized. The aforementioned considerations regarding initial incision and subsequent extensile options should be considered carefully in these instances.

Ascending Aorta and Transverse Arch

Injury to the ascending and transverse aortic arch is uncommon, but the exact incidence is unknown due to the lethality of these injuries. A widened mediastinum and cardiac tamponade are frequently associated with ascending aortic ruptures. Repair of these injuries most commonly requires a median sternotomy, cardiopulmonary bypass, and systemic heparinization. Management of the aortic tear may be primary or with a synthetic interposition graft. Special attention should be paid to the status of the aortic valve, which may be compromised and require repair or replacement. Injuries to the aortic arch may also require hypothermic circulatory arrest and associated antegrade and retrograde cerebral perfusion techniques to be employed.

Innominate Artery

Rupture of the innominate artery is the second most common thoracic arterial injury following blunt trauma. Innominate artery injuries can generally be repaired via a median sternotomy with a right cervical extension when necessary. Blunt injury typically involves the base of the innominate artery, and this is most expeditiously

Fig. 7.9 Placement of an ascending aorta to innominate artery bypass with oversewing of the innominate artery stump

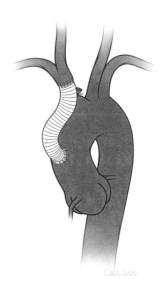

repaired with a bypass from the ascending aorta to the distal innominate artery, followed by over-sewing of the innominate stump (Fig. 7.9). Division of the innominate vein is occasionally required for exposure, and shunts or cardiopulmonary bypass is not often required.

Tip *Avoidance of the injured area until completion of the bypass improves the technical ease of repair.*

It is important to remember that blunt occlusions may not require emergent repair. Particularly when detected in a delayed fashion, revascularization must be based upon clinical scenario. Revascularization, particularly of an occlusion compromising carotid flow, may result in hemorrhagic conversion of existing ischemic lesions that may have already occurred. If no such cerebral ischemia has manifested, then collateral circulation has already proven sufficient to support adequate perfusion in the short term. In this setting, revascularization is indicated for persistent ischemic symptoms.

Left Common Carotid Artery

The surgical approach to injuries of the proximal left carotid artery mirrors that of the innominate artery—a sternotomy with a left cervical extension, if needed. With injuries of the left carotid origin, bypass graft repair is generally preferred over an end-to-end reanastomosis. The management of a carotid injury in the setting of neurologic disturbances is controversial. Generally, if the patient is evaluated soon after injury, revascularization is recommended because hypotension (rather than ischemic infarct) is the most likely cause of morbidity. Recently, traumatic carotid lesions have also been managed effectively with endovascular techniques. An endovascular approach may be especially useful for extensive lesions with involvement near the skull base, where challenges obtaining adequate proximal and distal vascular control through open approaches may result in increased morbidity. The goal of endovascular therapy in these settings is the elimination of a fistula, aneurysm, or stenosis while preserving native flow to the brain.

Subclavian Vessels

Injuries to the subclavian vessels are most commonly caused by penetrating mechanisms. When they can be obtained, the treatment of subclavian vascular injuries commonly benefits from preoperative imaging (generally CTA) for optimal incision planning. Injuries to the right subclavian artery are best addressed via a median sternotomy with a right cervical extension. Proximal control of left-sided subclavian injuries can be obtained via a left anterolateral thoracotomy. This incision can then be paired with a separate supraclavicular incision for distal control. These two incisions can be connected with a sternotomy to facilitate exposure, creating a "trap door" exposure. This incision should be used sparingly, however, as postoperative complications may be more common with this particular exposure. In addition, the second or third portion of the subclavian artery can usually be exposed without the need for clavicular resection or sternotomy.

Endovascular Repairs

As with BTAI, endovascular capabilities are increasingly being utilized to effectively treat vascular injuries to the vessels of the thoracic arch and thoracic inlet. Endovascular approaches to innominate, intrathoracic carotid, and subclavian arterial injuries have also been described in both blunt and penetrating traumas. Available data suggests that among appropriately selected patients, endovascular treatment is associated with improved outcome for injuries in these areas—which often represent challenging open exposures for control and repair.

In appropriate patients, endovascular repair should always be considered when developing a treatment plan. Defining "appropriate," however, has not been concretely defined outside of BTAI management. Despite this fact, if the patient is stable enough to tolerate CT imaging to adequately characterize thoracic vascular injuries—and appropriate expertise and equipment can be marshaled in an appropriate timeframe—discussion about the possibility of endovascular repair should be undertaken with appropriately qualified providers.

While this evidence suggests that endovascular repair modalities may have improved outcomes compared to open repair of a variety of thoracic vascular injuries during the initial hospitalization, it must be recognized that there remains a significant paucity of data on long-term outcomes. There remains a need to capture this data in order to better define if endovascular repair is to be considered definitive or simply a temporizing/damage control adjunct over the lifespan of a young trauma patient.

Another very important element of endovascular capabilities to consider is that the tools utilized in these emerging technologies need not be considered as definitive options only. Endovascular adjuncts can be used very effectively to improve the ability for injuries to be treated by open means. Endovascular occlusion balloons can be utilized to facilitate temporary proximal vascular control of thoracic branch vessels during open exposure and control. Covered stent grafts can be deployed to cover defects in large vessels and then be replaced in a staged fashion by open conduits if concerns about long-term outcomes of endografts remain. The ability to leverage technologies in this "hybrid" fashion may significantly improve outcomes following thoracic vascular injury.

Putting It All Together

Thoracic vascular injuries are challenging entities. In emergent settings, control of hemorrhage requires thoughtful consideration to the initial incision and a flexible approach to subsequent extension as required. Open repairs of proximal thoracic arterial structures may require the early engagement of cardiothoracic surgery partners, particularly if cardiopulmonary bypass is likely to be required.

Endovascular capabilities are emerging as viable alternatives to many thoracic vascular injuries—either as hybrid adjuncts to open repair or as definitive therapy. Though there remain many lessons to be learned with the use of these technologies, their use should be considered whenever possible. However, this employment requires the early activation of the required resources for their use.

Take-Home Points
1. The choice of initial incision is often a key decision—choose wisely but be prepared to extend as required.
2. Repair of the ascending and transverse aorta may require the use of cardiopulmonary bypass—activate those resources early if you need them in the emergent setting.
3. TEVAR is the primary repair modality for the vast majority of blunt thoracic aortic injuries.
4. Endovascular repair of thoracic great vessels may require origin coverage of adjacent vessel injuries—this is well tolerated for subclavian vessels but may require additional bypass at other locations.
5. Endovascular technologies are proving increasingly useful in the treatment of thoracic vascular injury—their potential application should at least be considered in the majority of injuries.

All bleeding eventually ceases. Guy de Chauliac

Chapter 8
Abdominal Vascular Hemorrhage: More than Just Clamp and Sew

David V. Feliciano

Introduction

Consider the following scenario:

A 47 year-old male sustains a shotgun wound to his torso. Persistent hypotension moves you into the operating room where you note massive hemorrhage from 4 holes within his distal abdominal aorta and inferior vena cava...

General Principles for Trauma Laparotomies

Skin preparation and draping for any laparotomy for abdominal trauma should extend from the chin to the knees bilaterally and to the operating room table laterally. This allows for the following: (1) extension into a median sternotomy, (2) the addition of an anterolateral thoracotomy, (3) distal control of an injury to the distal external iliac artery, and (4) retrieval of the greater saphenous vein as a vascular interposition graft.

After a xiphoid-to-pubis midline abdominal incision is made, all free blood, clot, and gastrointestinal or biliary contents are aspirated or swabbed out of the abdomen with laparotomy pads. With blunt trauma, the entire abdomen is rapidly inspected to localize sites of hemorrhage, hematomas, or gastrointestinal perforations. With penetrating trauma, the area of the knife or missile tract is inspected first followed by the rest of the abdomen.

D.V. Feliciano, MD (✉)
Battersby Professor Emeritus, Indiana University School of Medicine, Indianapolis, IN, USA

University of Maryland School of Medicine, Shock Trauma Center, Baltimore, MD, USA
e-mail: davidfelicianomd@gmail.com

© Springer International Publishing AG 2018
C.G. Ball, E. Dixon (eds.), *Treatment of Ongoing Hemorrhage*,
DOI 10.1007/978-3-319-63495-1_8

Approach to the Patient with Multiple Intra-abdominal Injuries Including an Abdominal Vascular Injury

Some patients with a retroperitoneal, mesenteric, or portal *hematoma* that is not rapidly expanding will be reasonably stable (systolic blood pressure > 90 mmHg). Preliminary control of perforations of the gastrointestinal tract is performed by rapid application of Allis, Babcock, or noncrushing intestinal (Glassman) or vascular (DeBakey, Cooley, Satinsky, Glover) clamps or by placing a staple line under the hole. The abdomen is then quickly irrigated with a saline solution containing a cephalosporin antibiotic. Finally, the surgeon changes contaminated surgical gloves and drapes before approaching the hematoma (see below).

Patients with *hemorrhage* are approached by eviscerating the transverse colon and small bowel as noted previously and covering these structures with two towels. Perforations in these structures are ignored until control and repair of the abdominal vascular injury are completed. After irrigation with a saline solution containing an antibiotic, the vascular repair or ligation is covered with retroperitoneal or mesenteric tissue or a viable pedicle of omentum and laparotomy pads soaked in the saline-antibiotic solution. Only then are the repairs of the gastrointestinal tract completed.

Obtaining Control of Injured Abdominal Vessels

Patients with retroperitoneal, mesenteric, or portal *hematomas* should have proximal and distal control with vascular clamps or vessel loops obtained before the hematoma is opened. One exception is when a massive retroperitoneal hematoma is present in addition to multiple other abdominal injuries. It is helpful to remember that the apex of the hematoma is over the hole in the abdominal vessel – the "Mt. *everest*" phenomenon. So, a very experienced abdominal vascular surgeon may enter this area directly, spread the hematoma manually, and grab the injured area with forceps or vascular clamps in the presence of major hemorrhage. This technique is rapid, works well with arterial injuries (venous injuries are often frayed and are stretched obliquely), mandates functioning suction devices, and is not for the fainthearted or inexperienced.

Patients with areas of *hemorrhage* should have finger or laparotomy pad compression applied to the area. Another unique option when the common or external iliac arteries and/or veins are bleeding rapidly is to have the surgeon *grab the vessels* with a hand after the pelvic retroperitoneum has been opened. Either laparotomy pad or temporary manual control of hemorrhage will allow the surgeon's assistant to obtain proximal and distal vascular control with DeBakey clamps. With injuries to the infrarenal inferior vena cava, common iliac vein, or external iliac vein, the time-honored technique of compression with sponge sticks around the area of injury will, again, temporarily control hemorrhage until vascular control is obtained. The insertion of an intraluminal balloon catheter is occasionally useful to control hemorrhage from larger abdominal vessels. This technique is most helpful when compression is ineffective, scarring from previous surgery delays obtaining proximal and distal vascular control, or the vascular injury is at a bifurcation (i.e., iliac vessel). The tip of the bladder catheter is inserted into the hole or tear in the vessel, and a 5-ml or 30-ml balloon is inflated and pulled tight against the edges of the injury. Another technique is the application of a row of Allis clamps to the sides of a large defect in a major vein of the abdomen. While much has been written about this technique to temporarily control venous hemorrhage over the past 25 years, it was described using "artery forceps" in 1916 during World War I! With hemorrhage mostly controlled by the row of clamps, venous repair is accomplished by a continuous over-and-over stitch as each clamp is removed. A less ideal option is to pass horizontal mattress sutures under the tips of the Allis clamps, but this will significantly narrow the area of repair.

Summary: Management of Abdominal Vascular Injuries

Management of abdominal vascular injuries is significantly more complex than peripheral vascular injuries. As noted in the Abstract, the obvious reasons are as follows: (1) patients are more often hemodynamically unstable, (2) tamponaded hematomas are larger, (3) the volume of hemorrhage is greater, (4) associated gastrointestinal injuries are common, (5) many vessels are more difficult to expose, and (6) many vessels have limited mobility when transected or resected.

For the trauma surgeon with limited experience in managing abdominal *arterial* injuries, the following brief summary will clarify the sections that follow:

Never ligate me, shunt me instead	Abdominal aorta Proximal superior mesenteric artery Common or external iliac artery
End-to-end anastomosis possible, otherwise insert graft	Renal artery Common or external iliac artery
Interposition graft mandatory	Abdominal aorta
Bypass graft mandatory	Proximal superior mesenteric artery
ok to ligate me	One internal iliac artery

For the trauma surgeon with limited experience in managing abdominal *venous* injuries, the following brief summary will clarify the sections that follow:

Never ligate me	Suprahepatic inferior vena cava
ok to ligate me for several hours, and then do delayed repair – might work	Suprarenal inferior vena cava
ok to ligate me (be prepared to treat sequelae!!)	Infrarenal inferior vena cava Renal vein Common, external, or internal iliac vein Portal, superior mesenteric, splenic, or inferior mesenteric vein

Midline Supramesocolic Hematoma or Hemorrhage

Hematoma or hemorrhage in this area may be caused by an injury to the diaphragmatic aorta, the supraceliac aorta, the visceral aorta, a visceral artery, and/or the suprarenal inferior vena cava. These are all large vessels, and patients surviving to reach the hospital will still have a significant mortality.

For the patient with a *hematoma*:

1. Perform the left medial mobilization maneuver to obtain proximal control of the aorta. Divide the lateral attachments of the descending colon, splenic flexure, spleen, and tail of the pancreas. If there is no extension of the hematoma to the left perirenal area, leave the kidney down. Finally, divide the attachments of the gastric fundus to the retroperitoneum.
2. The surgeon should slide the tips of the fingers of both hands across the retroperitoneum and elevate the left colon, spleen, tail of the pancreas, and gastric fundus to the midline. The assistant on the left side of the operating table assists using a Metzenbaum scissors.
3. Even with complete left-sided medial mobilization, the abdominal aorta is not visible because of overlying lymphatic tissue and the two celiac ganglia. Find the left crus of the aortic hiatus of the diaphragm. If the supramesocolic hematoma extends proximal to this, the injury is in the distal descending thoracic aorta or diaphragmatic aorta. Make a decision on whether it will be safer to perform a left anterolateral thoracotomy for cross-clamping of the descending thoracic aorta or stay in the abdomen. A hematoma inferior to this (may involve supraceliac or visceral aorta) can be approached as below.
4. With a decision to stay in the abdomen, place a Kelly clamp between the diaphragmatic aorta and the 2 o'clock position of the left aortic crus. This muscle is then divided radially with the electrocautery. The longer this incision is, the more the posterior left hemidiaphragm becomes distorted. If there is time, one marking suture on each side of the midpoint of the phrenotomy will make closure easier at the completion of the vascular repair or at a reoperation. A DeBakey aortic cross-clamp is applied to the diaphragmatic aorta to obtain proximal control.

For the patient with *hemorrhage*:

5. Apply an aortic compression device till the team is ready to proceed. Then, manually tear the lesser omentum longitudinally, and have the assistant retract the distal esophagus and stomach far to the left. Place your left hand through the omental tear till aortic pulsations (hopefully) are palpated. Attempt to insinuate your left second and third fingers inside the fibers of the aortic hiatus of the diaphragm. If this is not possible, divide the left aortic crus as noted in #4 above. Then apply a DeBakey aortic clamp vertically till the tips reach the vertebral bodies posteriorly and close the clamp to obtain proximal control at the level of the diaphragmatic aorta. This will substantially decrease any bleeding from an injury inferiorly, and dissection down the aorta should then be initiated.

Managing the vascular injury:

6. If dissection inferiorly on the anterior edge of the supraceliac aorta exposes an injury, repair a unilateral perforation with 4-0 polypropylene sutures, accepting some narrowing. Connect two adjacent perforations in the usual fashion, and close in a transverse or oblique fashion with the same suture. If loss of a portion of the wall without transection has occurred, sew in a thin-walled polytetrafluoroethylene (PTFE) patch with the same suture. Segmental resection will be necessary for some thru-and-thru or longitudinal perforations or a jagged near transection. There is no mobility of the supraceliac aorta because of the bilateral segmental lumbar arteries, so sew in an appropriately sized (#12–#16) woven Dacron or PTFE interposition graft using 4-0 polypropylene sutures. Remember, the edges of woven Dacron grafts fray easily after being trimmed, so take bigger bites of the graft than you would with a knitted Dacron graft. The needle holes in a PTFE graft will bleed like a sprinkler after declamping if an intraoperative coagulopathy is present, so avoid this graft when this complication has occurred. Leave the last few anterior sutures on the distal anastomosis loose to allow for proper flushing – proximal vascular clamp off to flush and then reapplied, distal vascular clamp off to flush air out under the anastomosis, proximal clamp off after sutures pulled tight, and one knot tied down. Finally, position and suture down a viable pedicle of omentum over both anastomoses and the graft to prevent a postoperative aortoduodenal fistula in these patients.

7. Further inferior dissection will expose the celiac axis, which is rarely injured. A major injury at its base mandates oversewing of the defect in the aorta and ligation of the branch vessels to control back-bleeding. An isolated injury to the proximal hepatic artery proper (angles toward the liver on the right), splenic artery (angles anteriorly), or the left gastric artery (easiest to visualize) is treated with ligation under "damage control" conditions.

8. Dissectioning inferiorly will almost immediately expose the origin of the superior mesenteric artery (SMA) as the celiac axis and SMA have a "V" conformation from the left lateral view (Fig. 8.1). A major injury at the base of the SMA (Fullen Zone I) on the aorta should be oversewn with 4-0 polypropylene sutures

Fig. 8.1 Left lateral appearance of visceral abdominal aorta after removal of celiac ganglia and lymphatic tissue. Note proximity of origins of celiac axis and superior mesenteric artery (Copyright, Baylor College of Medicine, 1980. Reproduced with permission; Baylor College of Medicine, 1986)

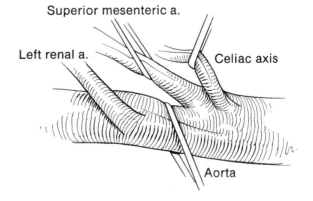

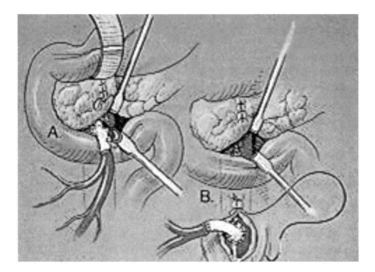

Fig. 8.2 A. Insertion of an interposition graft into the proximal superior mesenteric artery is contraindicated in the presence of an associated pancreatic injury. B. The proximal suture line should be on the lower aorta, away from the upper abdominal injuries, and should be covered with retroperitoneal tissue (Reproduced with permission from Accola K, Feliciano DV, Mattox KL et al.: Management of injuries to the superior mesenteric artery. *J Trauma*. 1986;26:313)

and the distal transected SMA ligated. With an injury to the proximal SMA in Fullen Zone II under the neck of the pancreas, divide the neck with an electrocautery for exposure and proximal control. When the injury is distal to the origin of the middle colic artery (Fullen Zone III), elevate the inferior edge of the pancreas for exposure and proximal control.

9. As previously noted, the proximal SMA should never be ligated in the modern era. When a very proximal injury is treated with oversewing of the aorta, there is no option to insert a temporary intraluminal shunt. As soon as other abdominal injuries are controlled, plan on doing an aorto-mesenteric bypass inferior to the mesocolon, etc. depending on the patient's temperature, hemodynamic status, and results of a TEG or ROTEM. With a significant injury to the SMA in Fullen Zone II or III, resect the injured segment and insert a #12 Fr. temporary intraluminal shunt to preserve arterial inflow to the midgut till a reoperation for the same bypass.

10. A bypass from the distal infrarenal abdominal aorta to the posterior SMA in the mesentery is described in other textbooks (Fig. 8.2).

11. An injury to the proximal renal artery is discussed in the section "Upper Lateral Retroperitoneum Hematoma or Hemorrhage."

12. An injury to the superior mesenteric vein (SMV) at the base of the mesentery of the small bowel or posterior to the neck of the pancreas will present with a midline supramesocolic or retromesocolic hematoma or hemorrhage, also. With a hematoma at the base of the mesentery, open the area directly to expose the

injured vessel, and grab this with a vascular forceps. Apply a large Satinsky vascular clamp around the injured area. Apply two DeBakey angled vascular clamps if the vein is transected, and ligate any mesenteric veins back-bleeding into the injured area. Approach a hematoma under the pancreas by dividing the neck with an electrocautery. This, of course, will release torrential hemorrhage if the injury is at the confluence of the SMV and splenic veins with the portal vein.

Your options for repair of the SMV include lateral venorrhaphy with 5-0 poly-propylene sutures, segmental resection and end-to-end anastomosis (push small bowel superiorly as anastomosis is performed to relieve tension), or insertion of a reversed autogenous saphenous vein graft. PTFE grafts will occlude in this location. Ligation is acceptable, but be prepared for postoperative distension of the midgut, need for a silo or vacuum-assisted device, splanchnic hypervolemia, and systemic hypovolemia.

13. For convenience, injury to the suprarenal inferior vena cava will be discussed in the next section.

Midline Inframesocolic Hematoma or Hemorrhage

Hematoma or hemorrhage in this area may be caused by an injury to the infrarenal aorta and/or infrarenal inferior vena cava (IVC), and the discussion on the suprarenal inferior vena cava is included, as well.

For the patient with a *hematoma* or *hemorrhage*:

1. A hematoma or hemorrhage at the base of the mesocolon should be approached as described in the previous Midline Supramesocolic section. Approach a hema-toma or hemorrhage which is truly inframesocolic by elevating the transverse mesocolon. Make a longitudinal incision in the midline retroperitoneum just inferior to the mesocolon, and dissect down to the crossover left renal vein. Dissect the infrarenal aorta just posterior to this down to the vertebrae, and apply a DeBakey aortic clamp. With a massive but still inframesocolic hematoma, the previously described direct approach through the highest point of the hematoma is acceptable for a senior surgeon.

Managing the vascular injury:

2. Once the aorta proximal to the area of injury is clamped, choose one of the repairs outlined previously for injuries to the supraceliac/suprarenal aorta. Should an extensive injury involve the bifurcation of the abdominal aorta, expose the common iliac arteries by extending the incision in the midline retroperito-neum. After applying DeBakey angled vascular clamps to the common iliac arteries or iliac bifurcations bilaterally, excise the injured bifurcation. Insert a woven Dacron aortic bifurcation graft by first completing the proximal aorta-to-graft anastomosis with 4-0 polypropylene sutures. After flushing, complete one

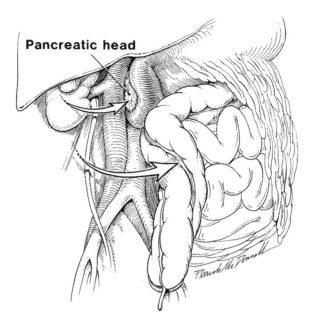

Fig. 8.3 Medial mobilization of right-sided intra-abdominal viscera except the kidney allows for visualization of entire infrahepatic inferior vena cava (Copyright, Baylor College of Medicine, 1981. Reproduced with permission)

graft-to-common iliac artery anastomosis using 5-0 polypropylene sutures. With the other graft limb clamped at its origin, flush the distal anastomosis of the first limb, and reestablish arterial inflow into one lower extremity. Then, complete the second limb-to-common iliac artery anastomosis.

Hematoma thought to be from an injured infrarenal IVC:

3. A primarily right-sided retroperitoneal hematoma elevating the cecum and ascending colon is likely to be from an injury to the inferior vena cava, and this is confirmed by ruling out injury to the infrarenal abdominal aorta as described above. After elevating the cecum and ascending colon (part of right-sided medial mobilization maneuver), open the lower midline retroperitoneum, and expose the IVC just superior to the confluence of the common iliac veins to allow for easy proximal clamping (Fig. 8.3). Perform a Kocher maneuver (remainder of right-sided medial mobilization maneuver), and make a separate incision in the superior to the right of the midline retroperitoneum several inches inferior to the liver, and expose the junction of the renal veins with the IVC. Before entering the hematoma, clamp the IVC just above the common iliac veins and just below the renal veins. Open the hematoma, and control an anterior hole in the IVC with a large Satinsky vascular clamp, row of Allis clamps, or the insertion of a balloon catheter.

Hemorrhage thought to be from an injured infrarenal IVC:

4. Apply laparotomy pad compression to the area of hemorrhage. Expose the IVC just superior to the common iliac veins and apply DeBakey aortic cross-clamp. If the compression is controlling bleeding, expose the justarenal IVC and apply an infrarenal cross-clamp as described above. If laparotomy pad compression is ineffective in controlling hemorrhage despite the presence of the inferior cross-clamp on the IVC, open the retroperitoneum directly over the area of hemorrhage. Control the area of hemorrhage with one of the previously described techniques or by applying pressure with sponge sticks until cross-clamps can be applied closer around the area of injury.

Managing the injury to the infrarenal IVC:

5. Close any solitary perforation or two adjacent perforations that have been connected in a transverse or oblique fashion with 4-0 polypropylene sutures. The needle on the 5-0 polypropylene suture is a bit small for IVC repairs. Close any separate posterior perforation by placing the starting knot, suture closure, and finishing knot in the OUTSIDE of the lumen. In a now stable patient, replace a loss of the wall of the IVC with a thin-walled PTFE patch or loss of a segment of the IVC with a ringed PTFE graft, etc. if the appropriate size can be found in the hospital. But, most patients with such extensive injuries or with a longitudinal split of the IVC in combination with "physiologic exhaustion" should have ligation of the infrarenal IVC. Before applying O-silk ties above and below the area of extensive injury, place cross-clamps around the area where the tie is to be placed so that it comes down on a collapsed IVC. Ligation is acceptable, but be prepared for postoperative distension of the lower extremities, a significant risk of the patient developing bilateral below-the-knee compartment syndromes and systemic hypovolemia.

Hematoma or hemorrhage thought to be from an injured suprarenal IVC:

6. Apply laparotomy pad compression to the area of hemorrhage. As previously described, incise the superior to the right of the midline retroperitoneum. Expose and apply an aortic cross-clamp to the infrarenal IVC, and apply DeBakey vascular clamps to the right and left renal veins at their junctions with the IVC. If there is space superior to the laparotomy pad compression and inferior to the liver, expose the infrahepatic IVC and apply another aortic cross-clamp. When no space for further dissection is possible, open the retroperitoneum over the area of injury, and accept temporary torrential bleeding until the actual perforation in the suprarenal IVC is controlled.

Managing the injury to the suprarenal IVC:

7. All repairs are similar to those described for the infrarenal IVC. Ligation will cause permanent renal failure in most patients. Avoid this unless the patient has a terminal arrhythmia such as ventricular fibrillation or has a cardiac arrest. If the

patient recovers miraculously in the SICU over the next 6 h without evidence of a coagulopathy, consider a return to the operating room for insertion of an appropriately sized ringed PTFE graft in place of the ligation.

Upper Lateral (Perirenal) Hematoma or Hemorrhage

Hematoma or hemorrhage in this area may be caused by an injury to the renal artery, renal vein, and/or kidney.

For the patient with a *juxtarenal hematoma*:

1. On the left side, perform left-sided medial mobilization and have the supraceliac aorta exposed to allow for cross-clamping if an injury to the proximal renal artery is found when the hematoma is opened.
2. On the right side, expose the supraceliac aorta through the lesser sac as previously described to allow for cross-clamping.

For the patient with *juxtarenal hemorrhage*:

3. As per right-sided juxtarenal hematoma above, as compression is applied to the area of hemorrhage.

For the patient with *perirenal hematoma or hemorrhage*:

4. Rather than the time-consuming older technique of placing a vessel loop around the ipsilateral renal artery (and left renal vein) at the midline, it is easier and faster to divide the retroperitoneum lateral to the kidney. Apply compression to the anterior kidney with one hand if there is hemorrhage, and elevate the injured kidney and/or hilar vessel out of the retroperitoneum with the other hand or with the assistant's help. Clamp actively bleeding hilar vessel once the kidney is fully elevated.

Managing the injury to the renal artery or vein:

5. If a penetrating injury has created a large defect in or transected the renal artery, quickly palpate for the presence of a normal-sized contralateral kidney. When one is present, perform an ipsilateral nephrectomy with separate ligations of the renal artery, vein, and ureter.
6. Should the other kidney be atrophic or absent, the patient will need to be reevaluated for a possible segmental resection of the renal artery. Then, one must decide whether a saphenous vein interposition graft is feasible. If not, call the vascular surgery team to perform an aortorenal artery bypass or the renal transplantation team to autotransplant the otherwise intact kidney to the pelvis.
7. When only a blunt thrombosis of the renal artery to the *one* normal kidney is present, consider a renal artery repair if less than 6 h have elapsed since the injury. Expose the ipsilateral renal artery at its junction with the aorta and place a vessel loop around it. Do the same at the renal artery distal to the hematoma. Then, divide the lateral retroperitoneum and fully mobilize the kidney. After

5000 units of unfractionated heparin are administered intravenously, resect the 2 cm or so area of the intimal tear. Perform an end-to-end anastomosis of the renal artery using 6-0 polypropylene sutures. Some centers place ice around the kidney when it is devascularized or infuse a renal perfusion solution distally after the segmental resection and before the anastomosis.

8. Approach a presumed perforation or tear in the renal vein (dark nonpulsatile hematoma in left juxtarenal area on or in right paracaval area or hemorrhage) by elevating the transverse colon and mesentery superiorly as previously described. To expose the crossover left renal vein, open the inframesocolic midline over the aortic pulsations and pass a vessel loop around the vein. Then, divide the retroperitoneum lateral to the left kidney and mobilize the kidney out of its bed so that the vein in the hilum is exposed. On the right side, perform a Kocher maneuver, divide the retroperitoneum over the juxtarenal IVC, and expose the right renal vein at its junction with the IVC. Again, pass a vessel loop around the vein and mobilize the right kidney out of its bed.

   As dissection proceeds on either side in the patient with a hematoma and sudden torrential hemorrhage is noted from a posterior perforation of the renal vein adjacent to the IVC, place a large Satinsky clamp around the renal vein-IVC junction. Be careful to avoid injury to the first posterior lumbar vein on the right which is adjacent to the right renal vein as this clamp is passed.

   Control of anterior perforations is with a Satinsky clamp, as well, though a row of Allis clamps should be placed if control is difficult to obtain.

9. Repair perforations with 5-0 polypropylene sutures accepting some narrowing. Uncontrolled hemorrhage despite attempts at clamping mandates ligation of the right renal vein at the IVC. This will, of course, have to be followed by a right nephrectomy at one of the "damage control" operations. On the left side, ligation of the renal vein at the junction with the IVC will still allow for venous outflow through the left adrenal and gonadal veins laterally. The function of the left kidney after this maneuver must be followed closely in the postoperative period.

Lateral Pelvic Hematoma or Hemorrhage

Hematoma or hemorrhage in this area may be caused by an injury to the iliac artery or branches, iliac vein or its branches, and/or the ureter.

For the patient with a *hematoma*:

1. After blunt trauma, *do not open* a lateral pelvic hematoma that is not expanding, is not pulsatile, and is unruptured. Only open the hematoma if the common or external iliac artery on one side is thrombosed.

2. After penetrating trauma, open the inferior retroperitoneum over the palpable aortoiliac bifurcation. Dissect out the ipsilateral common iliac artery, and pass a vessel loop around it. Do the same with the ipsilateral common iliac vein (these vessels are not adherent in young patients). Then, palpate the distal ipsilateral external iliac artery as it comes out of the pelvis and before it passes under the

inguinal ligament. Open the retroperitoneum over this, dissect out the external iliac artery and vein, and pass vessel loops around each. With four vessel loops in place, start dissecting from the superior loops inferiorly being careful to avoid the ureter. As bleeding is encountered from either the common or external iliac artery or vein, lift up the appropriate vessel loops, and apply DeBakey vascular clamps to the appropriate vessel.

For the patient with *hemorrhage*:

3. Apply laparotomy pad compression or the manual "grab" after the retroperitoneum at the site of hemorrhage is opened. Then, repeat the steps in #2 above. When hemorrhage is noted to be coming from the internal iliac artery, divide and ligate the overlying internal iliac vein for exposure. Uncontrolled hemorrhage from the inferior end of the IVC or proximal right common iliac vein may rarely require intentional temporary clamping and division of the overlying proximal right common iliac artery. Then, the aortic bifurcation is mobilized to the left for exposure of the venous injury (Fig. 8.4). On occasion, bilateral injuries to the iliac vessels from a transpelvic gunshot wound cause exsanguinating hemorrhage. Apply a large Satinsky clamp (or one each) around the aorta and IVC at the pelvic brim and another to each set of external iliac vessels (total pelvic vascular isolation described by Jon M. Burch, MD, Denver, CO).

Managing the injury to the iliac artery or vein:

1. In a "damage control" situation, resect the injured segment of the common or external iliac artery. Then insert an appropriately sized temporary intraluminal shunt till the reoperation.

Fig. 8.4 Intentional temporary division of the proximal right common iliac artery and mobilization of the aortic bifurcation to the right to expose injuries to the origin of the IVC or proximal right common iliac vein (Salam A, Steward M. *Surgery*. 1985;98:105)

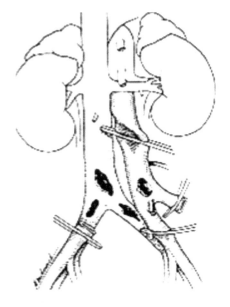

2. Without significant pelvic contamination by succus entericus or stool, all the standard repairs can be used for injuries to the common or external iliac artery. Choose lateral repair, segmental resection with an end-to-end anastomosis or interposition graft, or transposition of one common iliac artery to the side of the other using 5-0 polypropylene sutures. Divide and ligate a major injury to one internal iliac artery.

3. If there is *extensive* gastrointestinal contamination in the area of the arterial injury, be wary. A complex arterial repair is at risk for a postoperative arterial blowout. In the absence of support from a vascular surgeon, do the repair that is necessary. Then, mobilize a long pedicle of viable greater omentum and wrap it circumferentially around all sutures and/or graft used in the repair. With a vascular surgeon available, ligate the proximal uninjured common or external iliac artery with 5-0 polypropylene sutures. Then, cover the stump with uninjured pelvic retroperitoneum or, again, a long tongue of vascularized greater omentum. In a "damage control" procedure, perform an ipsilateral below-the-knee two-skin incision four-compartment fasciotomy to protect the now ischemic leg. After resuscitation in the SICU for 4–6 h, return the patient to the operating room for a crossover femoro-femoral bypass using an 8-mm-ringed PTFE graft. Remember, the crossover tunnel should NOT connect with the contaminated midline incision!

4. Repair a perforation in the common or external iliac vein with 5-0 polypropylene sutures placed in transverse or oblique direction. When a long narrowed segment results, when there is a longitudinal perforation, or when there is an extensive injury and "damage control" conditions, ligate the vein. Ligation is acceptable, but be prepared for a significant risk of the patient developing an ipsilateral below-the-knee compartment syndrome.

Portal Hematoma or Hemorrhage

Hematoma or hemorrhage in this area may be caused by an injury to the portal vein, common hepatic artery or branches, and/or the common bile duct.

For the patient with a *hematoma or hemorrhage*:

1. Place a DeBakey or Glover vascular clamp on the proximal porta hepatis. If there is a long enough porta, try to place another clamp across it at the liver. If unable, quickly dissect out and place a vessel loop around the common bile duct. Pull the duct vigorously to the patient's right side, and determine if the hematoma or hemorrhage is coming from the portal vein or hepatic artery. A perforation of the portal vein is elevated with a forceps, and a Satinsky clamp is placed under this. A perforation of the hepatic artery is managed the same, or proximal and distal bulldog vascular clamps are placed around it.

Managing the injury to the portal vein or hepatic artery:

2. Repair a perforation in the portal vein with 5-0 polypropylene sutures placed in a transverse or oblique direction. When a long narrowed segment results, when

there is a longitudinal perforation, or when there is extensive injury and "damage control" conditions, ligate the vein. Ligation is acceptable, but be prepared for all the sequelae previously described after ligation of the superior mesenteric vein.

3. Repair the common hepatic artery with lateral arteriorrhaphy or resection with an end-to-end anastomosis or saphenous vein interposition graft. Ligate an injured right or left hepatic artery as long as the ipsilateral portal vein branch is intact.

Summary

Saving the life of a patient with a major abdominal vascular injury depends on many variables as follows: patient's hemodynamic status, immediate operation, appropriate exposure and proximal and distal vascular control before entering hematomas, early control of hemorrhage, appropriate shunting or arterial repair, appropriate venous repair or ligation, and appropriate management of postoperative sequelae and complications. Using the techniques described, survival after injury to major abdominal arteries is 35–65% and after injury to major abdominal veins is 45–75%.

Take-Home Points
1. Abdominal vascular injuries are noted in only 5–10% of patients undergoing laparotomy for blunt trauma but in 20–25% of those with gunshot wounds.
2. The presence of injury to a major named abdominal vessel decreases survival by 35% in patients undergoing laparotomy for abdominal gunshot wounds.
3. A patient presenting with a major abdominal venous injury that is tamponaded by a hematoma will often have an admission blood pressure > 100 mmHg and a base deficit of only −5 to −10.
4. A patient presenting with a major abdominal arterial injury will often have an admission blood pressure < 100 mmHg and a base defect <−15.
5. A hypotensive patient undergoing laparotomy for a major abdominal vascular injury undergoes "damage control resuscitation" directed by thromboelastography (TEG, Haemonetics Corp., Niles, IL.) or rotational thromboelastometry (ROTEM, TEM INTERNATIONAL, GM6H, MUNICH, GERMANY).
6. Patients present with a contained hematoma, intraperitoneal bleeding, or a combination. Techniques of exposure will vary in some locations depending on the presentation. The five most common locations for hematomas or hemorrhage are as follows: (1) midline supramesocolic (Zone 1), (2) midline inframesocolic (Zone 1), (3) upper lateral retroperitoneum (perirenal/Zone 2), (4) pelvic retroperitoneum (Zone 3), and (5) porta hepatis/retrohepatic.
7. Associated intra-abdominal injuries are present in almost all patients, and unfortunately, many inpatients with penetrating wounds involve the gastrointestinal tract.
8. Most, but not all, major abdominal venous injuries can be treated with ligation under "damage control" conditions.

9. The celiac axis, a segmental mesenteric artery, or the internal iliac artery can be ligated if injured, but all other major named abdominal arteries should be shunted or repaired.

10. An open abdomen is not necessary after repair of a major abdominal vascular injury when bleeding has been controlled quickly by an experienced surgical team.

The most important clotting factor is the timely surgeon. Mosche Schein

Chapter 9
Liver Trauma Hemorrhage: The Bleeding Won't Stop!

Chad G. Ball and Elijah Dixon

Case Scenario

An 18-year-old male suffers a motocross crash. At the time of immediate laparotomy, your initial Pringle clamp fails to slow the retrohepatic hemorrhage that has become torrential. The anesthesiologist keeps pleading for help…

The problem with hepatic trauma always seems to be management of the hemodynamically unstable patient with a hemorrhaging high-grade liver injury. More specifically, these injuries can be difficult to expose, temporize, and/or repair for any surgeon who does not make their living in this region of the upper abdomen. These patients often present in physiologic extremis and therefore require damage control resuscitation techniques. Early recognition of their critical condition, as well as immediate hemorrhage control, is essential. Unlike the spleen and kidney, the liver cannot generally be resected in a rapid on-demand basis. Whether you are a trauma, acute care, or hepato-pancreato-biliary surgeon, these injuries will engage all your senses, test your technical skills, require the utmost focus, and demand great teamwork from you and your colleagues.

Patients with major injury because of blunt trauma or right upper quadrant penetrating trauma must undergo an immediate EFAST examination in the trauma bay to confirm the presence of large volume intraperitoneal fluid. This exam is repeatable and should be used to reevaluate patients in urban centers who present immediately following their injuries. Massive transfusion protocols as part of a damage control resuscitation must be initiated early during the patient assessment process.

C.G. Ball (✉)
Hepatobiliary and Pancreatic Surgery, Trauma and Acute Care Surgery, University of Calgary, Foothills Medical Centre, Calgary, AB, Canada
e-mail: ball.chad@gmail.com

E. Dixon
Hepatobiliary and Pancreatic Surgery, Division of General Surgery, Faculty of Medicine, Foothills Medical Centre, Calgary, AB, Canada

© Springer International Publishing AG 2018
C.G. Ball, E. Dixon (eds.), *Treatment of Ongoing Hemorrhage*,
DOI 10.1007/978-3-319-63495-1_9

If the patient rapidly stabilizes their hemodynamics, they should undergo an emergency CT scan of their torso. If they remain clinically unstable, they must be transferred to the operating theater without delay. Hemorrhage control is the dominant driver limiting survival. Collateral issues such as optimal intravenous access, imaging of other areas (brain, spine, bones), and fracture fixation are secondary issues.

The good news is that not all patients with liver injuries are actively dying secondary to hemorrhage. More specifically, in hemodynamically stable patients without CT evidence of a hepatic arterial blush, admission and close observation are warranted. In hemodynamically stable patients with a hepatic arterial blush, immediate transfer to the interventional angiography suite (or hybrid OR) is generally mandated. Hepatic angiography and/or portography with selective embolization is indicated with either autologous clot or absorbable embolization medium. In persistently hemodynamically unstable patients however, an immediate laparotomy is essential. More to the point, early recognition of a patient with ongoing hepatic hemorrhage, and immediate transfer to the operating theater, is crucial. Delays will lead to the loss of life.

The patient should be rapidly prepared and draped with available access from the neck to the knees. Vascular instruments and balloons must be open and at the ready within the theater. A midline laparotomy from the xiphoid process to pubic bone should be performed with three passes of a sharp scalpel. The peritoneal cavity should be packed in its entirety with laparotomy sponges for patients with blunt liver injuries. The falciform ligament can be left intact (especially in blunt trauma to the right lobe of the liver) to provide a medial wall against which to improve packing pressure. The right upper quadrant should be evaluated prior to any potential intraperitoneal packing for penetrating injuries. If hemorrhage continues, an early Pringle maneuver (clamping of the porta hepatis with a vascular clamp) is mandated. This is both diagnostic and potentially therapeutic. If bleeding continues despite application of a Pringle clamp, a retrohepatic inferior vena cava (IVC) or hepatic venous injury is likely (assuming that a replaced left hepatic artery is not the source of inflow occlusion failure). Critically injured patients in physiologic extremis do not tolerate extended Pringle maneuvers to the same extent as patients with hepatic tumors undergoing elective hepatic resection. Forty minutes represents the upper limit of viable. If the liver hemorrhage responds to packing, but continues to hemorrhage when unpacking is completed, they should be repacked and transferred to the ICU with an open abdomen once damage control of concurrent injuries is complete. Cover the liver with a plastic layer of sterile x-ray cassette material to avoid capsular trauma upon eventual unpacking. *Note: all major trauma procedures must be completed in less than 1 hour.* Return to the operating suite in patients with packed abdomens should occur in 48–72 h (assuming hypothermia, coagulopathy, and acidosis are corrected).

If the liver hemorrhage control is dependent on maintenance of a Pringle maneuver despite packing, call for senior assistance, mobilize the right lobe, and suture the IVC or hepatic veins with 4-0 Prolene on SH needles. These patients may also require total vascular occlusion of the liver. This technique involves complete occlusion of the infrahepatic IVC, suprahepatic IVC, porta hepatis (Pringle maneuver), as well as an aortic cross-clamp within the abdomen. If TVE is pursued without concurrent clamping of the aorta, the patient will typically arrest due to a lack of coronary perfusion. Prior to performing TVE of the liver, it is imperative to allow the anesthetic team to resuscitate the patient to the best of their ability to facilitate IVC clamping. We prefer to obtain suprahepatic IVC control within the abdomen in patients with a normal length of IVC inferior to the diaphragm. An alternate option includes access of the IVC within the pericardium itself as it enters the heart. This 2 cm length of IVC is easily accessible by opening the pericardial sac after dividing the central tendon of the diaphragm. Alternatively, it can also be accessed from the thorax if a thoracotomy has already been performed. Control of the infrahepatic IVC can be rapidly gained by opening the overlying peritoneum and bluntly encircling the IVC cephalad to the right real vein (i.e., no lumbar veins reside in this location above the renal veins).

Veno-veno bypass is also a theoretical option in some very specific scenarios but is rarely required if the patient can be adequately resuscitated to allow for IVC clamping. Furthermore, a lack of transplantation training in most trauma/general surgeons, and generally poor volume status of the patient, precludes expeditious use of this bypass.

In the case of central hepatic gunshot wounds or deep central lacerations where access and exposure are difficult, ongoing hemorrhage should be stopped with balloon occlusion. Either a Blakemore esophageal balloon or variant (red rubber catheter with overlying Penrose drain and two silk occlusion ties) is exceptional at stopping ongoing bleeding at the bottom of deep central hepatic injury tracts (including retrohepatic IVC injuries) (see the damage control chapter). Foley catheters of varying sizes are also helpful. These should be deflated approximately 72 h after the initial placement. If hemorrhage continues, they should be reinflated and left in vivo for 3 additional days.

Another excellent damage control option for major IVC disruption, portal vein injuries, and combined portal venous/hepatic arterial trauma is the use of temporary intravascular shunts (TIVS). TIVS is defined as a temporary synthetic conduit that ensures adequate inflow and/or outflow patency in the context of damage control for major vascular injuries. Although a large variety of tubes can be utilized as a TIVS (chest tubes (adult and pediatric), nasogastric tubes, carotid shunts, pediatric feeding tubes), they do not need to be heparin bonded. More specifically, TIVS typically fail for one of three reasons: (1) selection of a tube that is too small for the caliber of the disrupted vessel, (2) kinking of the tube itself, and (3) inadequate concurrent outflow (e.g., shunting of an iliac artery without ensuring adequate iliac venous outflow). IVC injuries in adults are usually best approximated with a 32- to 36-French chest tube. Portal veins are best shunted with a 22- to 26-French chest tube or large nasogastric feeding tube for small women. Hepatic arteries are best served by inserting pediatric nasogastric or feeding tubes. These TIVS may be locked into place with either silk ties or double-looped vessel loops and locking clips. The surgeon should choose the latter method in scenarios where maximizing the vessel distance is critical because the vessel will need to be further trimmed back beyond the silk ties when reconstruction is eventually attempted.

Vascular reconstruction following insertion of a TIVS should ideally involve an experienced HPB surgeon. The timing of this reconstruction will depend entirely upon the physiological and biochemical recovery of the patient. As soon as this is achieved by our critical care colleagues, the patient should return to the operating theater for repair. The surgeon must also ensure that a wide range of potential conduits is available and ready (saphenous vein, bovine pericardium, ringed and non-ringed PTFE). One superb conduit choice for IVC reconstruction following TIVS removal is bovine pericardium (or biologic mesh) that is fashioned into a tube of the appropriate size (usually wrapped around a bulb syringe with a single firing of a laparoscopic stapler to convert a sheet into a tube). This conduit performs very well in leaking/infected traumatic fields.

Although TIVS have revolutionized damage control trauma scenarios, the traditional damage control option for vascular trauma of ligation remains relevant. It is clear that based on a literature review of portal venous and superior mesenteric venous trauma, ligation of this vessel, rather than reconstruction, is often superior. This observation is likely multifactorial but almost certainly relates to surgeon unfamiliarity (i.e., time required to expose, control, and repair) with these vessels in anatomically hostile regions. Similarly, ligation of the IVC is also well recognized as a successful damage control maneuver (with postoperative leg elevation for 5 days and tensor bandage wrapping for 10 days).

Although unusual, patients with penetrating injuries to the hepatic artery will present as critically ill and may require ligation (assuming the portal vein is intact). Portal vein injuries should ideally be repaired with 5-0 or 6-0 Prolene once control is obtained. Clamps above and below the injury are essential for visualization. Alternate damage control options include TIVS with a small chest tube conduit or ligation (assuming the hepatic artery is intact).

If an atrial-caval shunt is ever contemplated, two experienced surgical teams (one for the chest and one for the abdomen) are essential to ensure both rapidity and efficiency. The decision to pursue this shunt must be made early in the exploration process. Unfortunately, these shunts rarely result in patient salvage in even the most experienced trauma centers. If a center and surgical team consider this maneuver to be part of their armamentarium for treating ongoing hemorrhage from retrohepatic injuries, a pre-stocked kit with all the necessary items must be readily available. Similar to utilizing TIVS and occlusion balloons, demanding rapid presentation of these instruments in the wee hours of the morning among a stressed clinical team in the context of a decompensating patient is likely to fail.

Allis clamps are also excellent for the initial control of venous hemorrhage. Do not be shy to call for an experienced assistant and/or elective hepatic surgeon. Topical hemostatic agents are also helpful. Fascial closure is ideal prior to discharge from the hospital. An institutional protocol to ensure fascial closure in complex patients is crucial.

Summary

It should be noted that although the published history of hepatic trauma is littered with descriptions of various technical maneuvers ordered in a hierarchical scheme, very few are relevant in context of modern trauma care. More specifically, packing of hepatic hemorrhage controls the vast majority of ongoing bleeding in critically ill patients. Selective uses of vessel ligation, parenchyma resection, and/or hepatic transplant remain less common strategies.

Ongoing hemorrhage from major hepatic injuries remains the most challenging of all intraperitoneal injuries due to issues with exposure, blood flow, and difficult technical repairs. Initiate damage control resuscitation and massive transfusion protocols early in your assessment. As with any damage control operation, all major components of the procedure must be completed within 1 h. Experienced surgeons will always have this clock ticking in the back of their minds. Flailing and indecision lead to prolonged operative times and patient demise. If diagnosis and therapy are rapid, patients who present in physiologic extremis because of major hepatic hemorrhage have a good chance of survival in the context of a prolonged hospital stay. Complications (bilomas, hepatic failure) must also be managed appropriately and without delay. Elective liver surgeons are usually experts in managing these issues, so call a friend!

Planned surveillance cross-sectional imaging (e.g., CT) is not required for major liver injuries (e.g., as opposed to splenic injuries). Repeat imaging should be based on deterioration in laboratory tests or patient symptoms.

The appropriate delay in time to return to physical/combat sports is debatable following major hepatic injury and associated hemorrhage. Despite a known 4–8-week hypertrophy response following elective hepatic resection, the time to regeneration and organ healing is unclear in the context of hepatic injuries.

Take-Home Points
1. Hepatic injuries are among the most challenging trauma scenarios for surgeons of all types.
2. Most bleeding hepatic injuries requiring operative therapy are treated with packing only.
3. TIVS and balloons can be a life-saving alternative to ligation for hepatic vascular damage control scenarios.
4. Prepare the patient for postoperative complications by selecting intraoperative life-saving procedures with the best chance of success and lowest risk of failure.
5. Involve an experienced HPB surgeon whenever possible to optimize outcomes in patients with hepatic trauma.

The only weapon with which the unconscious patient can immediately retaliate upon the incompetent surgeon is haemorrhage. William S. Halstead

Suggested Reading

1. Ball CG, Wyrzykowski AD, Nicholas JM, et al. A decade's experience with balloon tamponade for the emergency control of hemorrhage. J Trauma. 2011;70:330–3.
2. Feliciano DV, Mattox KL, Jordan GL Jr. Intra-abdominal packing for control of hepatic hemorrhage: a reappraisal. J Trauma. 1981;21:285–90.
3. Kozar RA, Feliciano DV, Moore EE, et al. Western trauma association/critical decisions in trauma: operative management of adult blunt hepatic trauma. J Trauma. 2011;71:1–5.
4. Lucas CE, Ledgerwood AM. Prospective evaluation of hemostatic techniques for liver injuries. J Trauma. 1976;16:442–51.
5. Pachter HL. Prometheus bound: evolution in the management of hepatic trauma- from myth to reality. J Trauma. 2012;72:321–9.
6. Pachter HL, Feliciano DV. Complex hepatic injuries. Surg Clin North Am. 1996;76:763–82.
7. Rozycki GS, Ochsner MG, Feliciano DV, et al. Early detection of hemoperitoneum by ultrasound investigation of the right upper quadrant: a multicenter study. J Trauma. 1998;45:878–83.

Chapter 10
Liver Resection Hemorrhage: Prevention is the Key!

Elijah Dixon and Chad G. Ball

Case Scenario

A 67-year-old female is undergoing an elective hepatic resection for a massive left-sided hepatocellular carcinoma. During the challenging outflow dissection, an injury to the main trunk of the left/middle hepatic veins occurs. The bleeding is audible and non-remitting…

The practice of liver surgery has changed dramatically over the past 20 years. When I was training as a resident and a hepatic resection was taking place, the case would not start until the blood products were in the room. Packed red cells were often transfused as the skin incision was made in anticipation of the blood loss to come. This is a marked departure from the typical rates of 10–20% rates of transfusion for major hepatic surgery now seen at expert centers.

Outcomes have improved for patients undergoing hepatic resection; this is a consequence of many key factors including improved knowledge of the intraparenchymal anatomy, improvements in the anesthetic techniques, the development of hepatobiliary surgery as a distinct specialty, and improvements in technologies that are used to assist in the parenchymal transection phase of hepatic surgery (energy devices and staplers). We have broken the chapter conceptually into two main phases, preoperative preparation and the surgery itself where it is further subdivided into six distinct phases: (1) opening and retraction/exposure, (2) preparation of inflow/outflow vessels, (3) parenchymal mapping and test clamping, (4) parenchymal division, (5) final hemostasis with biliary control, and (6) closure.

E. Dixon (✉)
Hepatobiliary and Pancreatic Surgery, Division of General Surgery, Faculty of Medicine, Foothills Medical Centre, Calgary, AB, Canada
e-mail: Elijah.Dixon@albertahealthservices.ca

C.G. Ball
Hepatobiliary and Pancreatic Surgery, Trauma and Acute Care Surgery, University of Calgary, Foothills Medical Centre, Calgary, AB, Canada

© Springer International Publishing AG 2018
C.G. Ball, E. Dixon (eds.), *Treatment of Ongoing Hemorrhage*,
DOI 10.1007/978-3-319-63495-1_10

Preoperative Preparation

All surgical procedures are best performed after careful preoperative planning; this is especially true for resectional hepatic surgery. The liver has complex internal anatomy based on inflow pedicles containing branches of the hepatic artery, portal vein, and biliary radicles all invested in Wallerian/Glissonian sheaths. These pedicles penetrate into the Couinaud segment they supply. In the vertical plane and running between the hepatic sections, the hepatic veins can be found. To safely perform hepatic surgery, the surgeon must have a complete and intimate knowledge of liver anatomy, both intraparenchymal anatomy and the external surface anatomy with special attention to the inflow and outflow vessels of the liver with an appreciation of potential variant anatomy. More than any other surgical discipline with the possible exception of neurosurgery, hepatic surgery requires that the surgeon constantly be thinking of the liver in reference to its three-dimensional structure with special attention to the inflow and outflow vessels running within the liver and their relation to the hepatic pathology in question. The relative position of these structures in relation to the surgeon is constantly changing as the surgeon frees the liver from its retroperitoneal attachments and brings the liver into the peritoneal cavity and rotates it to varying degrees from the patients' right to left on the axis of the inferior vena cava. Learning this anatomy is a lifelong pursuit that separates the master liver surgeon from the novice. Fortunately, the anatomic imaging currently available via CAT scanning and MR imaging is truly remarkable. Using a combination of the axial and coronal images, the surgeon can visualize the internal hepatic anatomy in ways not dreamed of 15 years ago. In addition, the reformatting of the images into 3-D reconstructions now allows the surgeon to truly see the anatomy of the liver in relation to the tumor in question.

The surgeon should run through the entire operation prior to starting the operation. Attention to those points in the operation that may be difficult should be the focus of this preoperative mental rehearsal. For every potential pitfall, the surgeon should have strategies in place to deal with all potential problems. In many cases specific measures should be taken to deal with potential pitfalls during the operation. Examples include placement of a Rumel tourniquet around the porta hepatis in most major hepatectomies, exposure of the infrahepatic vena cava in most major hepatectomies to allow caval clamping to lower the CVP if brisk hepatic venous bleeding is encountered, adjusting the incision used based on the planned procedure and the patient's body habitus, etc. The experienced liver surgeon will NEVER be surprised during a hepatic resection and will consequently avoid the potential pitfalls or deal with them when they arise without difficulty, thereby making it "look easy" most of the time.

The surgeon should ensure that the assistant has the appropriate level of skill for the resection. As opposed to many other surgical procedures, hepatic surgery at times truly requires a skilled assistant or second surgeon that can move the surgery forward on their own. There are scenarios and points in some hepatic cases where control of bleeding from the deep transection plane requires the hand of one surgeon to provide elevation of the liver from behind and either provide bimanual compression using the other hand or use of the sucker with the other hand to control the bleeding and improve visibility in the operative field. In these scenarios, the assistant needs to be able to definitively deal with the source of bleeding without close guidance by the surgeon (whose hands are tied up providing control, exposure, and optimization of the field). Many other surgical procedures can be completed almost entirely with one surgeon and a good retractor – this is not always the case in complex hepatic surgery. One does not want to be searching for a good assistant in the middle of the operation when brisk bleeding has already been encountered! A good chief resident, HPB fellow, or a second surgeon with experience in liver surgery are acceptable assistants.

The Operation

Opening and Exposure

The course and outcome of the surgery are largely dictated by decisions made regarding the choice of incision and the type of retraction system used. There are some general rules that usually hold true with regard to the type of incision used. First and foremost is flexibility with regard to the incision; many incisions are ideal for specific scenarios. Rigidly using one incision in all circumstances fails to take advantage of the optimal incision for a given operation and body habitus. For straightforward operations on the liver or the porta hepatis in patients with a relatively wide costal margin, either a bilateral subcostal or right subcostal incision with midline extension will provide excellent exposure. There are caveats to this statement. If the patient is barrel chested and/or very deep from anterior to posterior and a right-sided resection will be undertaken, then a midline incision from the xiphisternum to umbilicus with a direct lateral incision from the umbilicus to a point on the right flank midway between the costal margin and the iliac crest is ideal (right upper abdominal flap incision). This incision provides remarkable exposure to the right liver and the retrohepatic vena cava all the way up to the diaphragm. It is important that in contradistinction to most other incisions where the retractor is applied to the cut surface of the abdominal wall in this case, the right-sided abdominal flap is folded back on itself, and the retractor is placed on the costal margin hereby elevating the abdominal and chest walls anterior and cephalad. In cases where the costal margin is lengthy and acutely angulated in the midline, then either a long midline incision for left-sided resections or a right upper abdominal flap incision for right-sided resections provides excellent access. If another procedure is planned (synchronous colon and liver resections), then often a long midline incision is the ideal incision. In these cases, extension below the umbilicus provides surprisingly good access to the entire liver in conjunction with complete muscle relaxation. When opening and especially when dividing muscle, it is important to do this in a way that obtains complete hemostasis. Especially in complex multistep hepatobiliary operations with long operative times, the incision can contribute to a significant amount of blood loss over the course of a few hours if it is not completely hemostatic. The use of cautery along with careful attention to hemostasis will ensure that UNNECESSARY blood loss from the incision does not occur. THIS CANNOT BE OVEREMPHASIZED – all portions of the operation where blood loss is easy to prevent must be hemostatic if one hopes to have low operative blood loss. There are other portions of the operation where some blood loss is unavoidable. Lack of attention to detail and rushing will result in avoidable blood loss.

There are many different retraction systems available. Each has their own merits. Our system of choice is the Thompson (Farley) Retractor. Others that work well include the Omni and the Gomez. Despite differences in their use, they all provide exposure using similar principles. It is important to be familiar with one of these systems. The rigid retraction system should be mounted in such a way that it does not interfere with the surgeon and the assistant – this requires some distance from the operative field. The bar upon which the mountable blades are placed on should be high enough above the abdominal/chest wall that the costal margin can be elevated slightly and pulled cephalad – this is usually 1–1.5 handbreadths above the abdominal wall. The rigid bar should be placed 1.5–2 handbreadths away from the incision to allow adequate distance for cephalad retraction. It is important that the rigid bar is not mounted too high on the posts or it will create a deep "pit" which makes the surgery more difficult. Whenever possible, a complete ring of rigid fixation bars should be mounted around the operative field, ideally keeping the rigid bars 1.5–2 handbreadths away from the field. Mountable retractors should be used liberally to maximize exposure and free up the surgeon's and assistant's hands. Both costal margins should be retracted cephalad. The caudal half of the incision should be gently retracted caudal (if too vigorous, it fights against the cephalad retractors impairing exposure of the cephalad half of the liver). A deep malleable retractor should be used to gently retract the right kidney posterior and caudal. Sponges should be applied to the surface of all areas under retractor blades to increase traction. A second malleable blade on the left-hand side of the patient can be placed cephalad to the lesser curve of the stomach and just to the left of the caudate lobe and vena cava and used to retract the stomach and pancreas caudal. The surgeon should be unafraid to change the retraction setup multiple times in an operation if needed.

Preparation of Inflow/Outflow Vessels

A brief comment about the tempo of the operation is needed at this point. Aside from when some form of inflow/outflow occlusion is being used, there should be no "pressure" to proceed rapidly. Every step of the operation is simple if one knows the anatomy and potential pitfalls. Surgery should proceed methodically without rushing. As mentioned, care regarding hemostasis is important especially in the non-transectional phases of the surgery where all blood loss is avoidable. Proceeding in a methodical non-rushed fashion will usually result in the surgery proceeding quickly. Rushing and having too much bleeding are often in retrospect the first "hole" in the so-called Swiss cheese metaphor of the perfect storm where multiple holes line up in a way that leads to a very poor patient outcome. Doing things properly the first time prevents the surgeon from having to return to previous portions of the operation that need to be readdressed, ultimately slowing the operation, leading to greater blood loss, and sometimes starting the slow spiral toward a preventable bad patient outcome.

After proper retraction, mobilization of the liver is required. Our practice is to in general completely mobilize the liver for open operations. That is of course not always required, especially if left-sided resections are being undertaken. Any attachments between the gallbladder and the stomach, duodenum, or transverse colon are first divided. The ligamentum teres is divided between ties. In cases where there is a lot of preperitoneal fat near the midline, we will often excise this so that it does not obscure the view of the cephalad portion of the liver at this point in the operation. We then place a lap sponge behind the left lateral portion of the liver to protect the stomach posterior to it when we divide the left-sided cephalad ligamentous attachments of the liver. The triangular ligaments are divided on the cephalad side of the liver; the incision is made approximately 3–5 mm of the surface of the liver. This dissection is taken back until the hepatic veins are identified; gentle blunt dissection with the tip of the Yankauer sucker can facilitate this. Once identified, the left-sided attachments are completely divided over to the tip of segment 2. Segment 2/3 is then gently rolled to the right, and the stomach is retracted to the left, posterior and caudal; this exposes the lesser omentum which is divided under direct vision exposing the caudate lobe (care must be taken to identify an accessory or replaced left hepatic artery running through the lesser omentum). Division of these left-sided ligaments facilitates mobilization of the right lobe. The surgeon on the patient's left-hand side then rolls the right lobe up and out of the recesses of the right upper quadrant; while doing this, the left lobe is tucked into the left side of the abdomen. The diaphragm is grasped laterally and pulled gently to the right and slightly cephalad. Dividing its attachment to the liver approximately 3–5 mm off the liver is performed right up to the other area of mobilization which has previously exposed the right hepatic vein. This dissection is continued posterior and cephalad, which frees the liver from the retroperitoneum and delivers it into the wound. If dissection is not right on the liver, it is possible to generate bleeding from phrenic veins on the surface of the diaphragm. After the liver starts to rise forth out of the retroperitoneum, the point of tension will be the peritoneal attachments on the caudal side of the right lobe – the so-called rookie ligament (because it is commonly avulsed off the liver by the rookie surgeon). This should be divided under direct vision with the assistant providing gentle cephalad and anterior pressure on the caudal aspect of segments five and six along with countertraction on the right kidney and hepatic flexure. Division of this ligament continues from the lateral edge of the right lobe of the liver across to the infrahepatic vena cava. Once this has been divided, the right lobe starts to rise up out of the recesses of the right upper quadrant. Simultaneously the left lateral segment is "tucked" into the left upper quadrant; this facilitates rotation of the liver from right to left on the axis of the vena cava. Once the retroperitoneal attachments on the right are released, the liver is left attached only at the porta hepatis and the vena cava. After a decision has been made with regard to proceeding or not with the operation, vascular control can be obtained. If an extrahepatic approach to the vessels subserving the area to be resected is undertaken, this dissection and division can be carried out in the porta hepatis at this time. If nonselective inflow occlusion is used (Pringle maneuver), then our practice is to use an umbilical tape along with a Rob-Nel Catheter, which has been cut into thirds and is fashioned into a Rumel tourniquet. We have found that this type of occlusion is easily applied, results in complete interruption of inflow, and is not in the way (large vascular clamps often get in the way during the parenchymal transection). Prior to beginning the parenchymal transection, we will normally perform caval and hepatic vein dissection and isolation. If we are not performing total vascular exclusion, then we will typically dissect the liver off the vena cava and encircle the hepatic vein to be resected. We will also place an umbilical tape along the posterior transection plane and fix it to the drapes on the caudal and cephalad aspects of the wound in a modified "hanging liver" maneuver. This allows the surgeon to pull up on the tape during parenchymal transection and provide posterior compression to decrease blood loss. It also allows the surgeon to keep both hands working within the operative field. If TVE is used, then mobilization of the liver from the vena cava is not completed until after the posterior aspect of the retrohepatic vena cava is mobilized up out of the retroperitoneum. This is performed by dividing the right adrenal vein while rolling the right lobe "up and out" of the retroperitoneum dissecting from right to left along the back of the vena cava at the level of the divided adrenal vein. The caudate lobe rolls back around the vena cava on the left-hand side and can be felt as one dissects posterior to the vena cava. Cauterizing on the caudate lobe behind the cava will open a posterior window that will allow passage of a finger through the defect – the thumb can be used to roll the cava anterior while the index finger pulls the retroperitoneal tissue from left to right behind the cava. There should be no major branches in this plane as long as the surgeon stays cephalad to the renal veins. Umbilical tapes can be passed around the supra- and infrahepatic vena cava which makes it much easier to apply a vascular clamp when required later in the case.

As part of this phase of the operation, a decision should be made about the use of occlusive vascular techniques during parenchymal transection. If the resection will be done without TVE, then steps should be taken to ensure the CVP is as low as possible (<5 mmHG) to minimize hepatic venous bleeding. If during transection the CVP appears to be too high, then a partially or completely occluding vascular clamp across the infrahepatic IVC will usually drop the CVP adequately to allow safe liver surgery. If TVE is to be used, then the opposite is true; the patient must be volume loaded such that they will hemodynamically tolerate interruption of venous return to the heart from the liver.

Parenchymal Mapping and Test Clamping

The hepatic surgeon needs to be facile with intraoperative ultrasound. The surgeon should examine the liver carefully with the IOUS to assess the number and location of lesions and their relationship to major inflow and outflow pedicles/branches. The hepatic surface can be marked with cautery in such a way that clear margins can be obtained. The surgeon should not be afraid to use the IOUS during the resection as needed to confirm correct parenchymal transection trajectory.

Depending on the type of inflow/outflow occlusion to be used, now is the time to perform a test clamping trial to ensure adequate access to the pedicles and hemodynamic tolerance by the patient. As well, if ischemic preconditioning is to be used, this can be performed now. For cases where total vascular exclusion is to be engaged, a trial of clamping should be performed prior to transection to ensure that the patient will tolerate the clamping. The inflow clamp is applied first, followed by the infrahepatic caval clamp, and finally the suprahepatic caval clamp. Prior to application of the suprahepatic clamp, the liver can be gently massaged/squeezed to empty it of any remaining blood. The patient will experience a drop in mean blood pressure; this however should not be severe enough that the mean pressure is unacceptably low. If the pressure drop is prohibitive, then measures to ensure that the patient is properly volume loaded need to be undertaken. If the patient has not been adequately volume loaded and the preload on the heart is inadequate, then they will not tolerate clamping for the length of time required to perform a major hepatectomy. Options include placing the patient on veno-veno bypass or aborting the operation because of inadequate cardiac reserve.

Parenchymal Division

There are two key points to remember when the hepatic parenchyma is divided; first, never operate in a deep hole, and second, pay close attention to the pace of the operation. When performing open liver surgery, difficult bleeding can be made much worse if it occurs in a deep hole making control of the bleeding extremely difficult. A deep hole can be created by both the incision as discussed previously and the plane of transection through the liver. When the liver is split on a broad front, even significant hemorrhage can be controlled relatively easily by either direct suture control, vascular stapler division of major pedicles, or clip hemostasis. To ensure that a deep hole is not created, it is critically important to keep the resection in a horizontal plane (cephalad to caudad) as opposed to a vertical plane (anterior to posterior). Control of the inflow pedicle can be obtained using control of the porta hepatis or extrahepatic division of the vessels subserving the area to be resected; there is no need to quickly transect the anterior caudal aspect of the liver toward the hilar plate in a deep hole; rather the plate can be divided during major hepatectomy as one comes through the liver using a horizontal plane of resection from cephalad to caudad. Again, for segmental resections and non-anatomic resections, the same principle applies albeit with a shorter resection plane.

The pace of progress through the liver is largely dictated based on whether inflow occlusion is used. When the resection is performed under inflow control, warm ischemic time must be kept to a minimum. This dictates that the transection needs to be conducted quickly; only major pedicles should be controlled with ligature, clip, or vascular stapler. Small vessels and parenchyma should be divided quickly using Kelly fracture, ultrasonic dissection, or high-pressure water jet dissection. Oozing from small vessels often stops without control once the resected liver is removed or can be controlled using electrocautery, argon beam coagulation, or the bipolar sealing devices on the raw surface once the specimen has been removed. In contradistinction, transection without inflow control is best performed as quickly as possible all the while ensuring complete hemostasis during the transection phase. If good hemostasis is obtainable, then avoiding inflow occlusion and proceeding as fast as possible is the ideal hepatic resection – it avoids warm ischemia and avoids blood loss and all the negative consequences of autologous blood transfusion. The surgeon should control small vessels with cautery or other energy devices, move the resection site in such a way as to avoid the creation of a deep hole, and gently pack raw areas not being worked on with hemostatic substances like Surgicel or Gelfoam.

When bleeding is encountered, it can temporarily be controlled by gentle direct pressure ensuring the injury is not enlarged. Alternatively, the tape placed behind the liver in the plane of transection can be fixed to the drapes on the cephalad side of the liver and gently stretched caudal and anterior to provide gentle anterior compression from behind the liver (like placing a hand behind the liver and lifting it up anteriorly to minimize hepatic venous bleeding). If the bleeding is significant and arising from an inflow pedicle, then the transient use of inflow occlusion will allow improved visualization and control of the structures.

When performing major hepatic resections, especially when a large area of parenchyma will be divided or when the transection plane will be near the large named inflow/outflow pedicles, it is very important to have an assistant who is experienced and able to either expose and control the bleeding while the surgeon ligates it or vice versa. This is not something that should be arranged or called for during the case when the "trouble" has already started.

Final Hemostasis with Biliary Control and Closure

Once the specimen has been removed, the tendency to want to complete the operation forthwith needs to be held in check. This is the part of the operation where a too quick closure can lead to postoperative complications including the possibility of a return to the operating room. Careful meticulous attention to hemostasis is imperative, both raw surface and the area around the liver where the liver was dissected free from its ligamentous attachments. Once hemostasis has been achieved, attention can be directed to the search for any bile leaks. This is also critically important and requires a careful examination of the raw hepatic surface and any major inflow pedicles that were divided or dissected upon. If there is any concern, the pedicle should be carefully over sewn. If a vascular stapler was employed to divide the hilar plate where the plate is wide, sometimes the tissues can be "heaped up" in the stapler and have a tendency to leak (i.e. use a stapler used with adequate length).

The closure of the wound needs be performed in such a way that complete hemostasis is assured. Again, preventable blood loss should not be tolerated.

Conclusion

Hepatic surgery can now be performed safely with minimal blood loss in almost all cases. Important strategies to accomplish this include expertise in hepatobiliary surgery; careful anatomic planning of the conduct of the operation with attention to all potential pitfalls, ensuring good assistance and familiarity with a high-quality rigid retraction system; appropriate volume status manipulation to allow safe resection (low versus high CVP); parenchymal mapping so as to allow parenchymal-sparing surgery whenever possible; appropriate use of cautery and energy devices during the transection phase to minimize bleeding; transection in a horizontal plane (as opposed to a vertical plane which may create a deep, dark "hole"); generous use of hemostatic agents on the raw surface of the liver 'not being operated on' at the time; close attention to the appropriate tempo of the operation (vis-a-vis the use or lack thereof pedicle clamping and ischemia of the liver); posterior to anterior compression of the liver to decrease venous bleeding; and attention to detail while closing the patient and ensuring complete control of the biliary system.

By employing these techniques, the vast majority of patients should not require a blood transfusion.

Take-Home Points
1. Be the calmest person in the room when the bleeding starts.
2. Excellent exposure is king.
3. Attention to detail prevents most major hemorrhages.
4. Low central venous pressure is paramount to successful liver surgery.
5. Avoid the "deep, dark hole" during your parenchymal transections.

   The most common cause of post-operative coagulopathy is poor hemostasis. Mosche Schein

Chapter 11
Liver Transplantation Hemorrhage: Taking Bleeding to Another Level

Alan W. Hemming and Kristin L. Mekeel

> *Nothing we had done in advance could have prepared us for the enormity of the task. Several hours were required just to make the incision and enter the abdomen. Every piece of tissue that was cut contained small veins under high pressure that had resulted from obstruction of the portal vein by the diseased liver… His intestines and stomach were stuck to the liver in this mass of bloody scar. To make things worse, [the patient's] blood would not clot.*

> (Starzl 2003)

This quote from Tom Starzl describes the first human liver transplant on a 3-year-old boy with biliary atresia in 1963. As exemplified by this passage, liver transplantation creates the perfect storm for the development of massive, uncontrolled hemorrhage. To start, the pathophysiology of liver disease leads to portal hypertension and high-pressure venous collaterals that course through all of the abdominal tissue planes. Liver disease also results in severe coagulopathy from a lack of clotting factor synthesis and platelet sequestration in the spleen. The liver is located in the "surgical soul" of the abdomen, where the major vascular structures convene. Unique in its position and vascular structure, the liver has dual inflow of both the portal vein and hepatic artery and is intimately related to the inferior vena. Essentially, to successfully perform a liver transplant, you must extract the liver from a nest of high-pressure venous collaterals and all of the major vascular structures of the abdomen and then connect a new liver all in the background of severe coagulopathy. Every liver transplant surgeon can identify with cases that have been successful but required over 50 units of blood and even with occasional cases that reach the 100-unit mark but are generally not successful. It is a wonder that we are successful at this operation at all, and it is remarkable that most liver transplants are performed with 6–10 units of red cells with many tumor patients that have relatively less advanced liver disease requiring no blood at all.

A.W. Hemming • K.L. Mekeel (✉)
Department of Surgery, University of California San Diego, La Jolla, CA, USA
e-mail: kmekeel@ucsd.edu

© Springer International Publishing AG 2018
C.G. Ball, E. Dixon (eds.), *Treatment of Ongoing Hemorrhage*,
DOI 10.1007/978-3-319-63495-1_11

Significant progress has been made in liver transplantation since 1963 and Dr. Starzl's first liver transplant, but it is still an operation with the potential for substantial, ongoing blood loss and is not for the faint of heart. This chapter will review the anatomic and physiologic conditions inherent with liver disease that lead to bleeding and coagulopathy and review methods to control surgical and nonsurgical hemorrhage. Even if you are not or do not plan to be a liver transplant surgeon, lessons from liver transplantation can be used in any major trauma or surgical case.

Case Scenario

A 43-year-old female is undergoing a hepatic transplantation with a background history of hepatitis C cirrhosis. During the explant, the hemorrhage is torrential from a multitude of immense venous collaterals…

Anatomic and Physiologic Considerations

Portal Hypertension

With few exceptions, the pathophysiology of end-stage liver disease is similar across the spectrum of causative diseases. The hepatocytes sustain damage and die, creating fibrosis and scar; the remaining liver regenerates which leads to the shrunken, nodular liver typical of cirrhotic patients. The degree of fibrosis correlates with the severity of liver disease and portal hypertension. Because portal venous blood flows through the liver parenchyma on its way to the systemic circulation, fibrosis and scarring of the liver impede blood flow through the liver. Unable to drain through the usual route, the mesenteric venous system forms high-pressure collateral pathways of drainage around the liver. The most common pathways are the coronary vein to the esophageal plexus to the azygous, a recanalized umbilical vein, and through the inferior mesenteric vein to the superior rectal vein.

All liver transplant surgeons realize that the collateral pathways and varices extend far beyond the common routes. Almost every tissue plane in the abdomen is riddled with venous collaterals, under high pressure. These collaterals are evident in both the porta hepatis and the triangular ligaments, making mobilization of the liver difficult both due to bleeding and inflammation of these tissue planes. In addition, major collateral pathways between the splenic vein and the renal vein, the mesenteric veins and the iliac or femoral veins, and huge abdominal wall collaterals also exist (Figs. 11.1 and 11.2). It is imperative that the transplanting surgeon reviews imaging and identifies any potential major collaterals prior to transplantation, not only to prevent bleeding but to ligate in case of poor portal venous flow.

Because of these venous collaterals, many liver transplant surgeons do almost the entire dissection of the porta hepatis and triangular ligaments with the Bovie cautery and not a right angle or tonsil. Blunt dissection with spreading of the right angle or tonsil can transect venous collaterals and wreak havoc, leading to bleeding

Fig. 11.1 This figure demonstrates large intra-abdominal collaterals in a patient with cirrhosis and portal hypertension

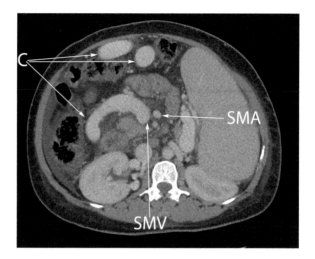

Fig. 11.2 This patient has large visible abdominal wall collaterals

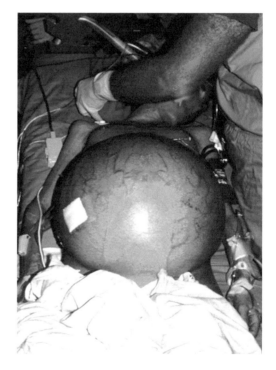

that is difficult to control because of the thin-walled, high-pressure nature of these collateral vessels. Instead, with some practice, the Bovie can be used to gently transect tissue with the heat and prevent bleeding from these small collaterals. Although this may seem counterintuitive, thermal damage to major vascular structures rarely occurs, and damage to vascular structures is actually less than what occurs with blunt dissection in a field of ongoing hemorrhage.

Coagulopathy

The liver is responsible for the production of all of the major clotting factors, with the exception for factor VIII and Von Willebrand factor Patients with end-stage liver disease can be both hypercoagulable and hypocoagulable because of the disordered factor production. It is not uncommon for a pretransplant patient to have a deep vein thrombosis or portal vein thrombosis prior to surgery from lack of synthesis of protein C, protein S, and other anticoagulant factors. However, in the operating room, the hypocoagulable state from lack of synthesis of procoagulant factors is the liver transplant surgeon's biggest enemy. Even after reperfusion of the donor liver, coagulopathy can persist especially when using marginal organs. It can take anywhere from 20 min to several hours for the liver to start producing coagulation factors. Patients with end-stage liver disease also are often severely thrombocytopenic, as the platelets are sequestered in the spleen as a result of portal hypertension.

The measurement of coagulopathy in the operating room is difficult. Traditional measures of coagulation are the platelet count, prothrombin time, prothromboplastin time, and fibrinogen. These labs do not accurately assess all of the intricacies of coagulation, in particular fibrinolysis and platelet function. In addition, the data is often inaccurate as there is a delay from when the labs are drawn to the results, and the state of coagulation is fluid and may have shifted in that time frame. Most liver transplant centers use a thromboelastogram (TEG) for accurate real-time intraoperative assessment of coagulation. The TEG monitors a sample of a whole blood as it clots and measures the speed and strength of clot formation. It can guide transfusions, factor replacement, and fibrinolytic therapy in a goal-directed manner and not only improves our ability to assess and correct coagulation deficits but also helps to not overcorrect and risk a possible thrombosis.

Veno-Veno Bypass

Historically, all liver transplant operations required intraoperative veno-veno bypass (also called portal-caval bypass) to decrease the peri-transplant portal hypertensive bleeding and hemodynamic instability from clamping in the inferior vena cava and decreasing preload. In veno-veno bypass, cannulas are placed in the femoral vein and portal vein, and venous blood is bypassed around the liver to a cannula in the axillary or jugular vein using a pump with a heparin-bonded motor (Fig. 11.3). Up until the portal vein is cannulated, there is still significant portal hypertensive bleeding; however, after the patient is placed on bypass d, the amount of portal venous bleeding decreases substantially, and hemodynamic stability can be maintained during hepatectomy and reperfusion (Fig. 11.4). Veno-veno bypass also allows for increased time for dissection and hepatectomy, which was particularly important when training fellows.

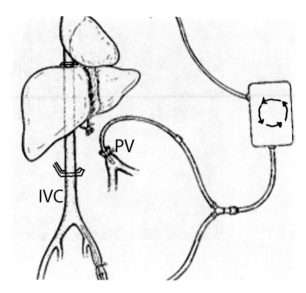

Fig. 11.3 This figure depicts veno-veno bypass. As noted in the text, cannulas are placed in the portal vein and femoral vein, so when the vena cava is clamped above and below the liver, blood is bypassed through a motor to the axillary or jugular vein

Fig. 11.4 This picture shows clamps on the suprahepatic and infrahepatic vena cava and the portal vein cannula in place for veno-veno bypass

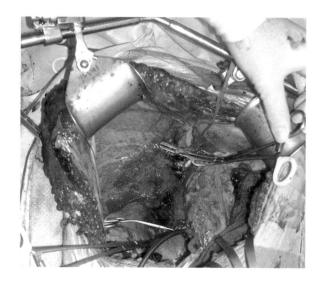

However, veno-veno bypass also had complications associated with it, including air embolism, venous thromboembolism, bleeding, seromas, and nerve injuries from the cannulas. In addition, it increased operative time and cost. In 1989, Tzakis published a paper describing "piggyback" liver transplantation, where the liver is dissected off the vena cava and a clamp is placed across the recipient hepatic veins

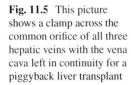

Fig. 11.5 This picture shows a clamp across the common orifice of all three hepatic veins with the vena cava left in continuity for a piggyback liver transplant

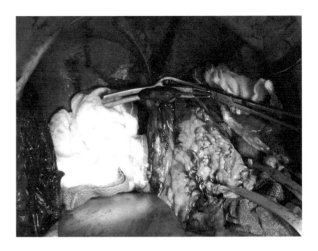

and not the vena cava (Fig. 11.5). The vena cava is left in continuity, and thus, there is less hemodynamic instability than when clamping the vena cava. Piggyback technique has been shown to reduce blood transfusion requirement despite operating in the portal hypertensive field. Veno-veno bypass is still the standard at some transplant centers; however, most programs now reserve bypass for surgically complex cases, in particular re-transplantation or a reoperative surgical field.

Surgical Bleeding

Major Vascular Structures

Surgical bleeding describes bleeding with a source that can be controlled with careful suture ligature, hemoclips, or other maneuvers. As the liver is closely associated with all of the major vascular structures of the abdomen, there is major potential for massive, specific bleeding from these structures that necessitates steady nerves and superior surgical skills.

The portal vein, and confluence of the portal vein, splenic vein, and superior mesenteric vein, has the potential to cause substantial grief during a liver transplant. These veins are often thin walled and tear easily. The trifurcation is also posterior to the neck of the pancreas making access nearly impossible. There can be multiple small portal vein branches that are directly into the portal vein just above the portal confluence. Dissection on the portal vein, in particular when dissecting the portal vein lower than the standard dissection to get below an area of stenosis or thrombosis, can result in avulsion of these small branches that subsequently result in torrential bleeding. Exposure and direct suture ligation are the best methods for control;

however, often, the bleeding is so brisk, and packing with hemostatic agents and allowing some inherent clotting to occur is often the first and best step. Care must be taken in the repair of these small veins, as the small injury can rapidly extend down the portal vein and be difficult to control if posterior to the pancreas.

If venous injury does occur, improving access if possible and careful suture ligature as not to amplify the problem are recommended. Clamping the portal vein can help control bleeding in the porta hepatis but will exacerbate any bleeding proximal to the clamp.

As mentioned above, approximately 30% of patients with liver disease undergoing liver transplantation have a partial or complete portal vein thrombosis. In some cases, these thromboses are acute and can easily be removed at the time of surgery, but in many cases, there is a chronic thrombus with evidence of cavernous transformation of the porta hepatis. Removing a chronic thrombus has the potential for serious and possibly unrecoverable venous injury. The portal vein is opened, and the thrombus is peeled from the vein wall, similar to an endarterectomy. This is completed to the neck of the pancreas; then a peon clamp is used to dislodge the clot from the trifurcation. If flow is reestablished, then the portal vein anastomosis continues as planned; if not, the surgeon must consider a venous interposition graft, using donor iliac vein, from the superior mesenteric vein. If venous laceration occurs, control may be difficult if not impossible if the laceration extends behind the pancreas. The only option is ligation with large sutures and placement of a venous jump graft from the SMV for inflow. This allows retrograde flow from the splenic vein down to the SMV, and both SMV and splenic flow will proceed through the venous jump graft to the allograft.

The hepatic veins and inferior vena cava are another potential source of substantial and potentially fatal bleeding during a liver transplant. In a standard liver transplant, the retro-hepatic vena cava is removed on block with explant and replaced with the donor liver vena cava. The risk for injury with caval replacement is the adrenal vein and even right renal vein when exposing the infrahepatic vena. If vascular injury occurs, direct exposure control and suture ligation of these are the preferred methods of control, but mass ligation may be necessary in the event of massive bleeding. In the piggyback method of liver transplantation, the liver is dissected off the infrahepatic vena cava ligating the short hepatic veins from the caudate to the vena cava. A large inferior hepatic vein draining segment 6 can also be present. This dissection is much more difficult in a cirrhotic patient, as the vena cava is often encased in vascular adhesions secondary to the inflammation from the liver disease and portal hypertension. Smaller short hepatic veins can be sealed and divided with a bipolar electrothermal device or hemoclips. Medium-sized short hepatic veins require silk ties or suture ligature. A large inferior hepatic vein is best controlled with a running suture or a vascular stapler.

It can be very challenging to expose the vena cava and major injury is possible. Exposure is the first consideration for caval dissection, and a large caudate lobe, as seen with Budd-Chiari syndrome and primary sclerosing cholangitis, can make exposure and dissection much more difficult. Transection of the portal vein earlier in the dissection is the best method to improve exposure; however, there is a risk of increasing bowel edema and ischemia especially if the recipient has not developed significant collaterals. Injury to the vena cava during hepatectomy can not only cause massive bleeding but can lead to air emboli which can be fatal.

The best way to control small hole in the cava is controlling the bleeding with your hand or forceps and then placing a large figure of eight 4-0 Prolene to close the hole. Small bites can tear the cava and lead to larger holes or tears which are much more difficult to repair. Large cava injuries are best controlled by clamping the vena cava and repairing the injury with a running suture. The cava can be clamped with a side-biting clamp or a series of allis clamps in some cases which keeps caval flow intact. Large injuries usually require clamping the entire vena cava above and below the injury to prevent exsanguination. Prior to clamping, advise your anesthesia team about the possibility for bleeding, air embolism, and hemodynamic instability with the injury and subsequent caval clamping. The cava can usually be repaired with a running Prolene suture. Large defects may need a patch to prevent stenosis, or consideration of converting to a caval replacement procedure is indicated if stenosis is inevitable. The base of the hepatic veins can also be a difficult place to control bleeding if injury occurs during liver transplant. In general the same principles outlined above need to be followed, but early clamping either of the hepatic veins themselves or of the vena cava is often the best way to get out of a difficult situation before it is too late. Do not underestimate bleeding from the vena cava or hepatic veins; it can quickly get out of control and lead to death of the patient.

In cirrhotics, the spleen can also be a source of massive hemorrhage during a liver transplant. Most cirrhotics have significant splenomegaly secondary to portal hypertension. The spleen can be damaged during dissection, especially of the left triangular ligament or with aggressive retractor placement. Even small rents in the congested spleen can lead to massive bleeding. The bleeding is always worse when the spleen is under high pressure from portal hypertension, can be substantially exacerbated during portal clamping, and may improve somewhat after reperfusion of the liver. Control of bleeding with the argon beam coagulator and topical hemostatic agents is the first line of defense. Partial splenorrhaphy is not indicated, and splenectomy should be a last resort, as it is a dangerous proposition in the face of portal hypertension, adhesions, and massive splenomegaly.

Nonspecific Bleeding

In liver transplantation, nonspecific bleeding is usually due to coagulopathy and is often referred to as the "you are screwed" bleeding because you can spend hours hoping the liver will start producing coagulation factors and trying to get the bleeding to stop.

Transfusion, Factors, and Antifibrinolytics

Transfusion of blood products remains the mainstay of the correction of coagulopathy during liver transplantation. Fresh frozen plasma is the most commonly used blood product after red blood cells and is given in a ratio of 1:1 or 2:1 similar to trauma patients to prevent factor depletion seen with the transfusion of PRBCs alone. Platelets are also given liberally, although not guided by absolute platelet count but by use of the TEG as outlined above. Cryoprecipitate is also used based on TEG profile and ongoing coagulopathy to replace fibrinogen with less volume required than would be needed with FFP.

However, in liver transplantation, ongoing bleeding continues after adequate factor replacement suggesting more complex coagulation abnormalities. Other commonly used products/factors include antifibrinolytics such as aminocaproic acid and tranexamic acid. Fibrinolysis is assessed by the TEG, and these products are started as an infusion during the transplant operation and continued for several hours post-transplant. Use of antifibrinolytics has been shown to reduce blood product use during liver transplantation. Protamine is also often used in liver transplantation. A significant dose (usually 30,000 units) of intravenous heparin is given to the donor and may contribute to a heparin type effect, in addition to the general overall coagulation factor deficit and heparin used in intraoperative irrigation.

Newer straight single factor and factor combinations have also been used frequently in liver transplantation. Recombinant factor VII is used most frequently and even though most studies have failed to show a benefit especially when cost is included in the analysis. Prothrombin complex concentrate (PCC) is also being used more frequently in transplantation. The complex contains factors II, VII, IX, and X as well as protein C and protein S. Earlier formulations were plagued by a high risk of thrombotic events, but the newer concentrates have a lower risk. Despite lack of evidence, these factors improve outcomes in liver transplantation, they are used when faced with ongoing hemorrhage due to coagulopathy, and all other treatments have been exhausted. Usually an immediate improvement in coagulopathy is noted, often enough to get the patient off the operating room table, but sometimes it is short lived and the coagulopathy recurs.

Surgical Devices

Multiple surgical devices can be useful during liver transplantation to decrease bleeding during and after liver transplantation. Standard Bovie electrocautery is a mainstay of liver transplantation, and used for dissection as described above. The argon beam is also used frequently. The argon beam uses a jet of argon gas to distribute radiofrequency current to a bleeding surface. It is best used for superficial surface bleeding. In liver transplantation, it is useful for all of the raw surfaces, especially portal hypertensive bleeding from small collaterals. A bipolar electrothermal vessel sealer is very useful for dissection and can be used in vessels up to 7 mm in width. It is useful for ligation of small- to medium-sized collaterals as well as the short hepatic branches off of the vena cava. The radiofrequency dissecting sealer is rarely used in liver transplantation, unless the graft is a split liver (either living or deceased donor) and there is a cut surface that needs coagulation. Large liver lacerations may also benefit from this device.

Topical Hemostatic Agents

There are three groups of topical hemostatic agents: agents that simulate coagulation (fibrin sealants), provide a matrix for coagulation (collagen, gelatin, and cellulose), and combinations of the two products (thrombin-Gelfoam, thrombin, and collagen). Fibrin sealants are usually a mixture of thrombin and fibrinogen that are mixed to form a glue. For most hemorrhage in liver transplantation, they have not been shown to be useful as the bleeding is too brisk and too broad to benefit from a small amount of fibrin sealant. However, in select cases, fibrin sealant maybe useful, for example, bleeding from needle holes or a small tear in a fragile anastomosis where suture repair may be treacherous.

Matrices, in particular cellulose and collagen, are the most commonly used products during liver transplantation. They provide a scaffold for coagulation, assisted by fibrin, thrombin, and other surface factors to help start the coagulation cascade. They are most useful for large raw bleeding surface areas to help spur on coagulation during ongoing bleeding and to help seal small holes in vessels or anastomoses were suture ligature may be perilous. Often large sheets of collagen or cellulose are used almost as a surgeon would use a sponge during the case, to help assist in coagulation. However, little evidence exists in liver transplantation that use of any topical hemostatic agents or use of one agent over another improves blood loss or outcomes after transplant.

Conclusion

In conclusion, liver transplantation is the perfect storm for hemorrhage. Portal hypertension, complex vasculature, and coagulopathy all come together and lead to the potential for massive hemorrhage and death. This chapter summarizes the advances over the last decades that led to fewer blood transfusions and a decreased mortality from liver transplantation and the methods liver transplant surgeons use to obtain to control ongoing bleeding from both surgical and nonsurgical sources. This information should be helpful to any surgeon operating on a cirrhotic patient or bleeding after a prolonged and difficult operation with coagulopathy from any source.

Take-Home Points

1. All liver transplant surgeons realize that the collateral pathways and varices extend far beyond the common routes. Almost every tissue plane in the abdomen is riddled with venous collaterals, under high pressure. These collaterals are evident in both the porta hepatis and the triangular ligaments, making mobilization of the liver difficult both due to bleeding and inflammation of these tissue planes.

2. Because of these venous collaterals, many liver transplant surgeons do almost the entire dissection of the porta hepatis and triangular ligaments with the Bovie cautery and not a right angle or tonsil. Blunt dissection with spreading of the right angle or tonsil can transect venous collaterals and wreak havoc, leading to bleeding that is difficult to control because of the thin-walled, high-pressure nature of these collateral vessels

3. Most liver transplant centers use a thromboelastogram (TEG) for accurate real-time intraoperative assessment of coagulation. The TEG monitors a sample of the whole blood as it clots and measures the speed and strength of clot formation. It can guide transfusions, factor replacement, and fibrinolytic therapy in a goal-directed manner and not only improves our ability to assess and correct coagulation deficits but also helps to not overcorrect and risk a possible thrombosis.

4. Exposure and direct suture ligation is the best method for control of small bleeding portal vein branches; however, often, the bleeding is so brisk, and packing with hemostatic agents and allowing some inherent clotting to occur is often the first and best step. Care must be taken in the repair of these small veins, as the small injury can rapidly extend down the portal vein and be difficult to control if posterior to the pancreas.

5. If venous injury to either the hepatic veins or portal veins does occur, improving access if possible and careful suture ligature as not to amplify the problem are recommended. Mass ligation is sometimes necessary as a last resort.

6. The best way to control small hole in the cava is controlling the bleeding with your hand or forceps and then placing a large figure of eight 4-0 Prolene to close the hole. Small bites can tear the cava and lead to larger holes or tears which are much more difficult to repair. Large cava injuries are best controlled by clamping the vena cava and repairing the injury with a running suture.

7. In cirrhotics, the spleen can also be a source of massive hemorrhage during a liver transplant. Most cirrhotics have significant splenomegaly secondary to portal hypertension. The spleen can be damaged during dissection, especially of the left triangular ligament or with aggressive retractor placement. Even small rents in the congested spleen can lead to massive bleeding. The bleeding is always worse when the spleen is under high pressure from portal hypertension, can be substantially exacerbated during portal clamping, and may improve somewhat after reperfusion of the liver.

8. In liver transplantation, ongoing bleeding continues after adequate factor replacement suggesting more complex coagulation abnormalities. Other commonly used products/factors include antifibrinolytics such as aminocaproic acid and tranexamic acid.

The blood bank is the surgeon's gas station. Mosche Schein

Chapter 12
Pancreas Resection and Pancreatitis Hemorrhage: Taking Years Off Your Life

Parsia A. Vagefi, Madhukar S. Patel, and Keith D. Lillemoe

Case Scenario

A 54-year-old male with chronic pancreatitis (chronic pain, biliary and duodenal obstruction) is undergoing a pancreaticoduodenectomy procedure. During the dissection of the portal vein off of the inflamed and scarred pancreatic head/uncinate, the vein is torn. The tear is propagated into a larger hole with further attempts at dissection. You are called to help…

Overview

Severe hemorrhage from pancreatic resection or as a sequela of pancreatitis is uncommon; however, when it does occur, it has been associated with significant morbidity and mortality when not recognized and intervened upon expeditiously. A thorough understanding of pancreatic anatomy and relationships to surrounding vasculature is necessary in order to determine the source of bleed and develop the most optimal plan for management. Although a surgical approach is favorable for control and reconstruction of vascular injury encountered during resection, nonoperative endovascular techniques are generally employed for treatment of bleeding encountered postoperatively or due to pancreatitis.

P.A. Vagefi
Liver Transplantation, Massachusetts General Hospital, Boston, MA, USA

M.S. Patel
General Surgery, Massachusetts General Hospital, Boston, MA, USA

K.D. Lillemoe (✉)
Department of Surgery, Massachusetts General Hospital, Boston, MA, USA
e-mail: klillemoe@hms.harvard.edu

© Springer International Publishing AG 2018   143
C.G. Ball, E. Dixon (eds.), *Treatment of Ongoing Hemorrhage*,
DOI 10.1007/978-3-319-63495-1_12

Relevant Pancreatic Anatomy and Relations

As a fixed organ of the retroperitoneum, the pancreas lies transversely between the C-shaped loop of the duodenum and the splenic hilum. Blood supply to the organ itself arises from the celiac trunk and superior mesenteric artery (SMA). Specifically, the parenchyma is supplied by arcades from the superior and inferior pancreatico-duodenal arteries as well as branches of the splenic artery, commonly including the dorsal pancreatic artery, great pancreatic artery, and caudal pancreatic artery. As the vasculature of the pancreas is highly variable among patients, detailed review of axial imaging acquired in the arterial and portal venous phase is important prior to undertaking any intervention.

Anatomically, the pancreas is divided into five parts (the head, uncinate process, neck, body, and tail), each having distinct vascular relations that are important to consider when planning an operation as well as an approach for hemorrhage control. Generally, the pancreaticoduodenal arcades run along the anterior and posterior surface of the organ in the head region, whereas the major arteries and veins supplying the body and neck lie posterior to the pancreatic duct, with the veins typically being superficial to their correlating arteries. Moving from right to left, important vascular relations to consider by anatomic region of the pancreas are as follows:

Head: As mentioned, the anterior and posterior pancreaticoduodenal arcades run on superficial and deep surfaces of the pancreatic head, respectively. Notably, the posterior surface of the pancreatic head lies atop the right renal hilum as well as the inferior vena cava which receives the right gonadal vein on its anterior surface.

Uncinate process: The uncinate process is positioned anterior to the inferior vena cava and aorta and posterior to the superior mesenteric artery and superior mesenteric vein (SMA and SMV, respectively). In this position, in the sagittal plane, the left renal vein lies above the uncinate process and the third portion of the duodenum below. Importantly, the uncinate process is supplied by short vessels from the SMA and SMV. Additionally, it may be traversed by an accessory or replaced right hepatic artery.

Neck: The superior mesenteric vessels run posterior to the neck of the pancreas, where the portal vein is formed at the confluence of the SMV and the splenic vein. A number of small veins drain into the SMV or portal vein (PV), typically on their lateral aspect. At the inferior border of the pancreatic neck, the inferior pancreaticoduodenal vein as well as right gastro-omental vein can often be identified draining into either the splenic vein, SMV, or portal vein. Also related to the neck of the pancreas is the dorsal pancreatic artery which branches off from the proximal splenic artery.

Body: the aorta and SMA takeoff lie in the longitudinal plane, posterior to the body of the pancreas. The splenic vessels lie orthogonally, coursing in a tortuous pattern, transversely along the superior aspect of the body into the pancreatic tail. The body of the pancreas also lies anterior to the left renal hilum, kidney, and adrenal gland.

Tail: the splenic vessels continue posterior to the tail of the pancreas which abuts the splenic hilum.

Pancreatic Resection

Hemorrhage related to pancreatic resection can occur during or after pancreatic surgery and, depending upon etiology, is managed by open, endovascular, or endoscopic therapy.

Intraoperative Hemorrhage Control

Hemorrhage may be encountered during any of the critical steps of pancreatic resection, stressing the importance of knowing not only the relevant anatomy but also techniques in optimizing exposure so that bleeding can be controlled and repair performed. Clear communication with the anesthesiology team and nursing staff is critical throughout the procedure so that adequate resuscitation can be performed and additional access acquired if necessary. Specifically, since venous dissection and the potential for bleeding can occur early in the course of the procedure, it is important to confirm the immediate availability of cross-matched packed red blood cells. Although considerable attention to hemostasis is warranted in all operative procedures, the increasing use of neoadjuvant therapies for locally advanced pancreatic cancers in a significant proportion of patients undergoing pancreaticoduodenectomy for cancer should heighten the awareness of the surgeon during these cases as the tissue planes are often more difficult to define and are more prone to bleeding [8]. If significant bleeding is encountered, initial maneuvers to obtain hemostasis include applying direct manual pressure until anesthesia is able to adequately resuscitate the patient and is prepared for attempts at surgical repair. Despite such bleeding appearing dramatic, over-resuscitation with excessive crystalloid should be avoided to prevent the development of small bowel edema which may hamper reconstruction. If bleeding is encountered after kocherization of the duodenum, manual pressure can be applied by placing the fingers of the nondominant hand behind the pancreatic head with the thumb anterior to the pancreatic parenchyma so as to compress the vessels in between [4]. In order to obtain definitive control, exposure should be optimized, sometimes requiring early pancreatic transection and/or specimen removal so that proximal and distal control can be obtained. If the source of vascular injury is apparent, vascular clamps may be temporarily applied until repair is performed. Approaches to hemorrhage control of commonly injured vessels during pancreatic resection as well as considerations for hemorrhage encountered during laparoscopic and hybrid approaches are discussed below.

Inferior Vena Cava (IVC) or Renal Hilum

Inadvertent injury to the IVC or renal hilum vessels may be encountered during kocherization of the duodenum. As these structures are deep, manual pressure can be applied through use of long surgical sponge sticks fashioned on ring forceps.

Fig. 12.1 Intraoperative
image following
pancreaticoduodenectomy
with resection and primary
reconstruction of the
superior mesenteric vein
(*SMV*) (anastomosis –
white arrow). *Panc*
pancreas, *SV* splenic vein,
PV portal vein

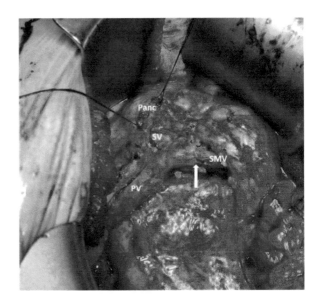

After pressure tamponade of ongoing bleeding, the injury may be localized and
venous injury primarily repaired with monofilament polypropylene suture.

Superior Mesenteric Vein

Dissection and exposure of the SMV may lead to significant, difficult-to-control
bleeding as this vessel has numerous venous tributaries. Hemorrhage from the SMV
is often from avulsion of venous branches associated with the gastrocolic trunk as it
receives the right gastro-omental vein and middle colic vein. The fragile nature of
the vein, often worse after neoadjuvant therapy, can result in a small tear being
extended during attempts at control or repair. In this situation, manual pressure is
once again advised, with precise over-sewing of the injury once identified. Temporizing with atraumatic (Allis) clamps or surgical clips is often necessary to control
bleeding during the actual repair. It is important to clearly determine the specific site
of the bleeding, as due to the small size of the SMV, blind attempts at hemostasis
may result in increased damage or result in impaired mesenteric venous drainage
secondary to narrowing of the vessel. To the latter effect, once hemostasis is
achieved, if there is significant narrowing of the luminal diameter of the vessel,
consideration should be given for resection of the affected segment with primary
reconstruction (Fig. 12.1).

Portal Vein

Dissection of the common bile duct (CBD) during pancreaticoduodenectomy puts the posterior lying PV at risk for injury. Particularly, in patients with preoperative CBD stenting, there should be heightened awareness by the surgeon as reactive inflammation may lead to a more challenging dissection. Division of the common bile duct as well as medialization of the hepatic artery after ligation of the gastro-duodenal artery (GDA) may help increase exposure of the PV for repair. Additionally, risk for injury of the PV also exists during creation of the retropancreatic tunnel behind the neck of the pancreas. If bleeding is encountered during this step of the operation, packing of gauze in the retropancreatic space to pressurize the tunnel formed along the anterior border of the PV and SMV should be considered. A vessel loop can then be placed around the supra-pancreatic PV and infra-pancreatic SMV which are both typically well dissected prior to creation of this tunnel. If significant bleeding persists, an additional tourniquet can be placed around the body of the pancreas for splenic vein control. As mentioned above, transection of the pancreas may be necessary in order to increase exposure for PV repair.

Once bleeding is controlled and exposure optimized, the portal vein can be primarily repaired with polypropylene suture or with patch repair when approximately >30% of the lumen is compromised using either autologous vein (internal jugular, left renal, splenic, or greater saphenous vein) or bovine pericardial patch [11]. In cases in which portal vein reconstruction is needed, either due to iatrogenic injury or after planned portal vein resection due to adherent tumor, circumferential dissection of the portal vein toward the hilum, as well as circumferential mobilization of the SMV, may allow for primary end-to-end reconstruction without the need for graft. Additional length for reconstruction may be obtained with division of the splenic vein (Fig. 12.2). In cases where interposition is needed (i.e., when greater than 5 cm of the portal vein is removed in the authors' experience), prosthetic grafts can be utilized for bridging; however, it should be noted that these grafts are associated with a higher rate of postoperative thrombosis, and thus, primary reconstruction or use of autologous vein grafts is preferred [11].

Superior Mesenteric Artery

Prior to removing the transected and dissected pancreatic head specimen, SMA injury may occur as the right lateral branches of the artery to the uncinate as well as the inferior pancreaticoduodenal artery are ligated. If bleeding is encountered during this step, manual pressure can be applied by lifting the mobilized specimen upward and applying digital pressure to the bleeding vessels [4]. Proximal as well as distal control should subsequently be obtained so that primary repair of the SMA with polypropylene suture can be performed.

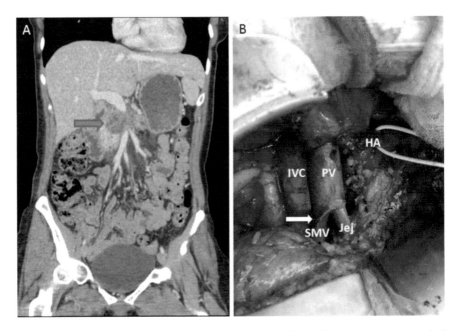

Fig. 12.2 (**a**) Preoperative computed tomography image acquired with portal venous protocol of a patient with a large pancreatic adenocarcinoma (*blue arrow*) showing encasement of the superior mesenteric vein (SMV) and splenic vein (SV) confluence. (**b**) Following completion of neoadjuvant chemoradiation, the patient underwent pancreaticoduodenectomy involving resection and reconstruction of the portal vein (*PV*) utilizing a double-barrel vascular reconstruction technique for the SMV and jejunal branch (anastomosis – *white arrow*). Despite resecting a large segment of the vein, a tension-free primary reconstruction was achieved by full mobilization of the PV toward the hilum, division of the splenic vein, and full mobilization of the SMV and jejunal branch. *IVC* inferior vena cava, *HA* hepatic artery, *Jej* jejunal vein

Hepatic Artery

Similar to the PV, the hepatic artery can be injured during the dissection of the CBD while performing pancreaticoduodenectomy or during ligation of the GDA. Arterial injuries should be repaired with polypropylene suture. As opposed to an accessory right hepatic artery which may be ligated if injured, damage to the common, proper, or a replaced hepatic artery should be repaired primarily after proximal and distal control is obtained. Right hepatic artery ligation, however, can lead to liver necrosis and subsequent infection, especially if the patient has infected bile from preoperative biliary stenting. An intraoperative Doppler ultrasound can be used to help further delineate any anomalies in arterial anatomy encountered as well as evaluate repairs performed on an injured hepatic artery.

Splenic Vessels

Injury to the splenic artery and splenic vein may be encountered during distal pancreatectomy and is managed by ligation, as opposed to repair. For patients with splenic vein thrombosis (SVT) or occlusion from extrinsic tumor compression of the splenic vein, extreme care should be taken during dissection due to the presence of significant collateralization and development of varices. In these situations, obtaining proximal control of the feeding splenic artery, as it abuts the superior aspect of the pancreas, may help decompress these collaterals if bleeding is encountered. In the case of splenic vein injury, control of the supra-pancreatic PV and infra-pancreatic SMV may be inadequate in achieving hemostasis as there are multiple tributaries that run along the course of this vessel that require individual ligation.

Considerations for Laparoscopic or Hybrid Approaches

Although laparoscopic pancreatic resection has been shown to have lower mean operative blood loss and intraoperative transfusion requirement compared to open resection [7], a low threshold for conversion should be maintained in cases of bleeding that are difficult to control in procedures performed through a minimally invasive approach. Initial attempts at hemorrhage control should include the temporary increase in insufflation pressure to provide tamponade of venous vessels in patients that can tolerate decreased cardiac preload. In situations where it is thought that bleeding may be controlled laparoscopically, insertion of additional 5 mm trocars may help facilitate exposure and subsequent repair [4]. In cases where bleeding persists and attempts of hemorrhage control are inadequate, the procedure should immediately be converted to open. Direct pressure on the site of presumed hemorrhage should be applied with a laparoscopic instrument during open conversion so as to decrease the amount of blood lost during the conversion process.

Postoperative Hemorrhage Control

Postpancreatectomy Hemorrhage (PPH) Classification

Bleeding occurring after pancreatic resection, also known as PPH, has been defined by the International Study Group of Pancreatic Surgery (ISGPS) based on three parameters: onset, location, and severity [17]. In this scheme, onset may be either early (within 24 h of operation) or late (after 24 h), location is either intraluminal or extraluminal, and severity is classified as being either mild or severe (transfusion requirement of more than three units of packed red blood cells, drop of hemoglobin greater than or equal to 3 g/dl, or need for invasive treatment). Grades of PPH are subsequently given as either A, B, or C based on these factors as well as the clinical impact of the bleeding. Importantly, this classification of PPH helps frame the discussion on management.

PPH Management Considerations

Early PPH resulting in hemodynamic instability which is not responsive to resuscitation should be emergently taken to the operating room for exploratory laparotomy. Early PPH is typically a technical complication and is often due to persistent bleeding from resection surfaces, sites of enteric anastomoses, drain site bleeds, or secondary to underlying coagulopathy. Principles discussed above for control of bleeding during pancreatic resection are thus applicable. For staple line or anastomotic bleeds encountered on reoperation, control can be obtained with surgical clips, interrupted sutures, or low-voltage cautery. Those patients with suspected early PPH who respond to resuscitation can be monitored closely while maintaining a low threshold for further evaluation and return to the operating room if clinical condition worsens.

In patients with late PPH, either hemodynamically stable or unstable, localization of the bleed is critically important in determining a treatment approach. A very low threshold for workup should be in any patient with even a small amount of hematemesis or blood in surgical drains, as these signs may represent a "sentinel bleed" proceeding a major hemorrhagic event. Immediate CT angiography with arterial and portal venous phase should be obtained in patients suspected to be bleeding. In cases of extraluminal PPH secondary to erosion of major visceral vessels and subsequent formation of pseudoaneurysms either by extrinsic compression from drains placed at the time of resection, intra-abdominal abscess, or postoperative pancreatic fistula (POPF), immediate digital subtraction angiography should be performed with either stenting (Fig. 12.3) or coil embolization (Fig. 12.4) [2, 16]. Although both methods of transcatheter angiographic intervention are effective, covered stents often offer the advantage of preserving hepatic artery blood flow [16]. If angiographic intervention is unsuccessful in controlling extraluminal bleeding or when associated POPFs in the setting of hemorrhage cannot be adequately controlled, reoperation should be performed with completion pancreatectomy considered in these later cases.

For hemodynamically stable patients with intraluminal PPH, the differential is broad and includes anastomotic bleeding (from the pancreatic stump of the pancreaticojejunostomy or pancreaticogastrostomy as well as from the gastroenteric or enteroenteric suture lines), hemobilia (from preoperative transhepatic biliary drainage), ulceration, or gastritis. Upper endoscopy can be performed with caution in these patients during the first 10 postoperative days and may be useful in evaluating the stomach as well as the accessible anastomotic sites. In patients with hemobilia, biliary stents may be placed and upsized. In those with recurrent or persistent bleeding, angiography with intervention should be pursued and, if unsuccessful, followed by reoperation which may result in completion pancreatectomy. Of note, in patients

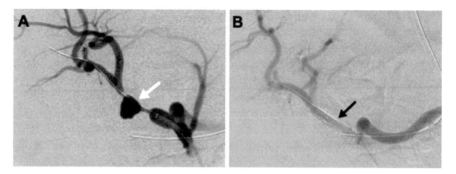

Fig. 12.3 Diagnosis of postpancreatectomy hemorrhage (PPH) caused by gastroduodenal artery (GDA) pseudoaneurysm without extravasation (panel **a**, *white arrow*) managed by placement of three covered stents (panel **b**, *black arrow*) for exclusion

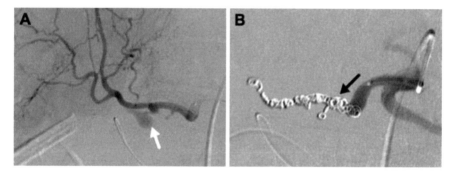

Fig. 12.4 Diagnosis of postpancreatectomy hemorrhage (PPH) caused by gastroduodenal artery (GDA) pseudoaneurysm with extravasation (panel **a**, *white arrow*) managed by coiling from the level of the proper hepatic artery, across the GDA stump, and to the level of the common hepatic artery (panel **b**, *black arrow*)

appearing to have intraluminal bleeding in the setting of ongoing POPF, a high suspicion of pseudo-intraluminal hemorrhage should be maintained (i.e., extraluminal bleeding manifesting as hemorrhage from the gastrointestinal tract), and these patients should proceed expeditiously to interventional angiography, similar to those with extraluminal PPH.

Pancreatitis

Bleeding in the setting of pancreatitis is most often due to either pseudoaneurysm formation of the pancreatic or peripancreatic vessels or as a sequela of SVT which may lead to variceal bleed. Pseudoaneurysms occur more commonly in chronic pancreatitis as compared to acute pancreatitis, at a frequency of 6–17% [18].

Differing from patients with pseudoaneurysms after pancreatic resection who often present with gastrointestinal bleeding or blood in the surgical drain associated with hypotension, those with pseudoaneurysms in the setting of pancreatitis often present with increased "crescendo" abdominal pain, different in quality from their typical pancreatitis pain [19]. The release of proteolytic and lipolytic pancreatic enzymes in the setting of inflammation as well as erosion of vessels from the extrinsic compression, ischemia, and elastolytic action of pancreatic pseudocysts is felt to cause pseudoaneurysm formation [9]. Once formed, these pseudoaneurysms are at subsequent risk of free rupture into the abdomen, retroperitoneum, or into surrounding structures such as pseudocysts themselves or other hollow viscera. With regard to SVT, it occurs at a frequency of approximately 14% and results in left-sided sinistral portal hypertension leading to associated variceal bleeding in 12.3% of patients [6]. Further discussion about the management of arterial bleeding due to pseudoaneurysms, venous bleeding secondary to SVT, and hemorrhage during or after pancreatic debridement for necrotizing pancreatitis is presented below.

Arterial Bleeding Due to Pseudoaneurysms from Chronic Pancreatitis

The source of arterial hemorrhage in patients with chronic pancreatitis is most commonly from pseudoaneurysms of the splenic artery (40%), GDA (30%), or the pancreatic duodenal (20%) arteries [13]. Patients with pancreatitis and suspected arterial hemorrhage should undergo urgent CT angiography of the abdomen with arterial and portal venous phase imaging. In addition to providing details about the pancreatic and peripancreatic vasculature, CT imaging provides an assessment of the underlying degree of pancreatitis. Those patients that are hemodynamically unstable despite adequate resuscitation should receive open intervention with proximal and distal ligation of the bleeding vessels and use of techniques for hemorrhage control as described above. Of note, in the setting of ongoing active pancreatitis, an open approach is technically challenging and associated with increased morbidity and mortality due to increased difficulty of dissection as well as tissue friability. Alternatively, in the hemodynamically stable patient, digital subtraction angiography should be pursued, and endovascular coil embolization should be used to exclude arterial pseudoaneurysms. In order for this method to be successful, upon completion of transcatheter intervention, arterial occlusion both proximal and distal to the area of pseudoaneurysm should be achieved as the vast number of collaterals around the pancreas will otherwise continue to feed the area of concern and may lead to recurrent bleed. Although less morbid than open surgery, angiography with embolization is not without complication which, in addition to access site morbidity and contrast-related challenges, includes potential for ischemia, infarction, or abscess formation of distal organs due to nontarget embolization [19]. In experienced centers, image-guided thrombin injection of pseudoaneurysms associated with pancreatitis provides an additional approach for cases that are not amenable to angiographic management either due to nonvisibility (secondary to delayed filling from a narrow neck), prior surgical clipping, or difficult anatomy [10]. In this technique, either CT, transabdominal ultrasonography, or endoscopic ultrasonography can be used as the imaging modality [10].Once adequate visualization is achieved, the pseudoaneurysm is punctured under image guidance, and aliquots of 100 international units (IU) of thrombin are injected until the pseudoaneurysm becomes non-enhancing or without color filling on color Doppler ultrasound.

Venous Bleeding Due to Splenic Vein Thrombosis from Chronic Pancreatitis

Venous complications of pancreatitis are typically secondary to significant inflammation leading to abscess or pseudocyst formation which causes thrombosis of the adjacent splenic vein. This, in turn, leads to formation of gastric varices which may bleed and result in massive hemorrhage. Patients presenting with gastrointestinal bleeding in the setting of pancreatitis are typically worked up with an upper gastrointestinal endoscopy in order to identify the source of bleeding and subsequent axial imaging. On CT angiography, it is important to differentiate SVT from portal hypertension as management of bleeding from these two distinct etiologies differs. On CT scan, SVT typically presents with low attenuation of the splenic vein, normal enhancement of the portal and superior mesenteric vein, and without evidence of umbilical vein recanalization [14]. As patients with SVT may develop silent collaterals that do not result in gastric or gastroesophageal varices, presence of SVT alone on imaging is not an indication for intervention, and observation is the preferred management strategy in asymptomatic patients [5, 6, 12]. However, in patients with bleeding secondary to SVT or symptomatic hypersplenism, splenectomy is the definitive treatment of choice as it results in decreased inflow to venous collaterals and subsequent decompression of associated varices [1, 5, 6, 15]. In patients who are initially unable to tolerate an operation, a second-line alternative to decrease collateral inflow is splenic artery embolization. As this technique may be complicated by the subsequent formation of splenic abscesses, a second stage of the procedure consisting of splenectomy is ultimately recommended [13].

Bleeding During or After Pancreatic Debridement

In patients with necrotizing pancreatitis, bleeding may be encountered during operative debridement. Preventative measures include using blunt instead of sharp debridement technique and performing selective debridement of only obviously necrotic material. In the case intraoperative bleeding encountered, control is usually blind as the source is often not easy to visualize. For bleeding occurring after debridement as identified through increased sanguineous drain output, emergent CT angiography with embolization is preferred. As minimally invasive approaches such as video-assisted retroperitoneal debridement (VARD) become increasingly used as part of a step-up approach to managing infected pancreatic collections, caution should be maintained not only intraoperatively during which bleeding which may be temporized with packing but also after the procedure, at which time delayed bleeding may require emergent CT angiography with intervention. Lastly, for cases of massive hemorrhage and significant metabolic derangement, it is important to note that the institution of damage control resuscitation (DCR) may be necessary [3]. In addition to immediate hemorrhage control by surgical or angiographic means, DCR protocols typically include the use of early blood transfusions, reduced crystalloid resuscitation, correction of hypothermia and acidosis, and delayed abdominal fascial closure in those warranting an operation [3].

Conclusions

Hemorrhage during pancreatic resection and as a sequela of pancreatitis requires prompt diagnosis and intervention. Significant bleeding encountered intraoperatively should be managed with direct pressure tamponade, optimization of vascular exposure, obtainment of proximal and distal control, and subsequent repair. Although postoperative hemorrhage in the hemodynamically unstable patient often warrants operative exploration, the majority of significant bleeds after pancreatic resection due to pseudoaneurysm formation should be managed with digital subtraction angiography and coil embolization or stent graft exclusion. Similarly, in arterial hemorrhage as a sequela of pseudoaneurysm formation in the setting of pancreatitis, endovascular techniques can be used successfully in most cases. In SVT leading to variceal bleed, however, splenectomy remains the first line of therapy. Lastly, as management of hemorrhage in all situations relies on a coordinated approach between members of the ancillary staff, anesthesia, surgery, and radiology teams, clear communication is paramount in order to most appropriately care for the patient suffering from pancreatic hemorrhage.

Take-Home Points
1. Initial maneuvers to obtain hemostasis for hemorrhage encountered during pancreatic resection include applying direct manual pressure until anesthesia is able to adequately resuscitate the patient and the team is prepared for attempts at surgical repair.
2. For definitive control, exposure should be optimized, sometimes requiring early pancreatic transection and/or specimen removal so that proximal and distal control can be obtained.
3. In cases in which portal vein reconstruction are needed, circumferential dissection of the portal vein toward the hilum, as well as circumferential mobilization

of the SMV, may allow for primary end-to-end reconstruction without the need for prosthetic grafts which carry a higher rate of postoperative thrombosis.

4. Damage to the common, proper, or a replaced hepatic artery should be repaired primarily after proximal and distal control is obtained.
5. A low threshold for conversion should be maintained in cases of bleeding that are difficult to control in procedures performed through a minimally invasive approach.
6. Early postpancreatectomy hemorrhage (within 24 h of operation) resulting in hemodynamic instability which is not responsive to resuscitation should be emergently taken to the operating room for exploratory laparotomy.
7. The majority of significant late bleeds (after 24 h of operation) after pancreatic resection due to pseudoaneurysm formation should be managed with digital subtraction angiography and coil embolization or stent graft exclusion.
8. Bleeding in the setting of pancreatitis is most often due to either pseudoaneurysm formation of the pancreatic or peripancreatic vessels or as a sequela of splenic vein thrombosis which may lead to variceal bleed.
9. Patients with pancreatitis and arterial hemorrhage should undergo digital subtraction angiography and endovascular coil embolization.
10. For bleeding secondary to splenic vein thrombosis, splenectomy is the definitive treatment of choice.

It's not the blood loss you can see that will get you, it's the blood loss you can't see.
Mosche Schein

References

1. Agarwal AK, Raj Kumar K, Agarwal S, et al. Significance of splenic vein thrombosis in chronic pancreatitis. Am J Surg. 2008;196(2):149–54.
2. Ansari D, Tingstedt B, Lindell G, et al. Hemorrhage after major pancreatic resection: incidence, risk factors, management, and outcome. Scand J Surg. 2016;106(1):47–53.
3. Ball CG, Correa-Gallego C, Howard TJ, et al. Damage control principles for pancreatic surgery. J Gastrointest Surg. 2010;14(10):1632–3; author reply 1634.
4. Ball CG, Dixon E, Vollmer CM, et al. The view from 10,000 procedures: technical tips and wisdom from master pancreatic surgeons to avoid hemorrhage during pancreaticoduodenectomy. BMC Surg. 2015;15(1):122.
5. Bradley EL 3rd. The natural history of splenic vein thrombosis due to chronic pancreatitis: indications for surgery. Int J Pancreatol. 1987;2(2):87–92.
6. Butler JR, Eckert GJ, Zyromski NJ, et al. Natural history of pancreatitis-induced splenic vein thrombosis: a systematic review and meta-analysis of its incidence and rate of gastrointestinal bleeding. HPB (Oxford). 2011;13(12):839–45.
7. Croome KP, Farnell MB, Que FG, et al. Total laparoscopic pancreaticoduodenectomy for pancreatic ductal adenocarcinoma: oncologic advantages over open approaches? Ann Surg. 2014;260(4):633–8; discussion 638–40.
8. Ferrone CR, Marchegiani G, Hong TS, et al. Radiological and surgical implications of neoadjuvant treatment with FOLFIRINOX for locally advanced and borderline resectable pancreatic cancer. Ann Surg. 2015;261(1):12–7.

9. Flati G, Andren-Sandberg A, La Pinta M, et al. Potentially fatal bleeding in acute pancreatitis: pathophysiology, prevention, and treatment. Pancreas. 2003;26(1):8–14.

10. Gamanagatti S, Thingujam U, Garg P, et al. Endoscopic ultrasound guided thrombin injection of angiographically occult pancreatitis associated visceral artery pseudoaneurysms: case series. World J Gastrointest Endosc. 2015;7(13):1107–13.

11. Glebova NO, Hicks CW, Piazza KM, et al. Technical risk factors for portal vein reconstruction thrombosis in pancreatic resection. J Vasc Surg. 2015;62(2):424–33.

12. Lillemoe KD, Yeo CJ. Management of complications of pancreatitis. Curr Probl Surg. 1998; 35(1):1–98.

13. Mallick IH, Winslet MC. Vascular complications of pancreatitis. JOP. 2004;5(5):328–37.

14. Marn CS, Edgar KA, Francis IR. CT diagnosis of splenic vein occlusion: imaging features, etiology and clinical manifestations. Abdom Imaging. 1995;20(1):78–81.

15. Sakorafas GH, Sarr MG, Farley DR, et al. The significance of sinistral portal hypertension complicating chronic pancreatitis. Am J Surg. 2000;179(2):129–33.

16. Wellner UF, Kulemann B, Lapshyn H, et al. Postpancreatectomy hemorrhage–incidence, treatment, and risk factors in over 1,000 pancreatic resections. J Gastrointest Surg. 2014;18(3):464–75.

17. Wente MN, Veit JA, Bassi C, et al. Postpancreatectomy hemorrhage (PPH): an International Study Group of Pancreatic Surgery (ISGPS) definition. Surgery. 2007;142(1):20–5.

18. Woods MS, Traverso LW, Kozarek RA, et al. Successful treatment of bleeding pseudoaneurysms of chronic pancreatitis. Pancreas. 1995;10(1):22–30.

19. Zyromski NJ, Vieira C, Stecker M, et al. Improved outcomes in postoperative and pancreatitis-related visceral pseudoaneurysms. J Gastrointest Surg. 2007;11(1):50–5.

Chapter 13
Pancreas Trauma Hemorrhage: So Much Trouble from this Small Organ

Chad G. Ball and Elijah Dixon

Case Scenario

A 20 year-old male sustains a sword wound. During initial exploration, you identify a transected inferior vena cava, lacerated suprapancreatic portal vein and a near complete transection of both the right kidney and the pancreatic head. The patient's physiology defines hostile…

Ongoing hemorrhage from either the hepatobiliary or pancreatic regions continues to daunt even the most experienced surgeon. Despite the widespread centralization of elective pancreatic surgery to high-volume centers, pancreatic trauma remains uncommonly common and requires a rapid and thoughtful approach from all surgeons.

Although the blood flow throughout the pancreatic gland is impressive, the dominant source of hemorrhage associated with pancreatic trauma remains the mesenteric venous structures that surround it. More specifically, the superior mesenteric, portal, inferior mesenteric, and splenic veins are the primary culprits. Although the anatomy of the portal and superior mesenteric veins is relatively constant, the insertion point of the inferior mesenteric vein can vary dramatically (i.e., insertion into the splenic and/or portal veins). It is also generally stated that the portal vein does not possess any branches arising from its anterior surface (i.e., immediately posterior to the pancreatic neck). As with many dogmatic anatomic comments, this "rule" is not infrequently broken. The presence of large venous tributaries from the portal vein into the head and uncinate of the pancreas is absolute however. The largest of

C.G. Ball (✉)
Hepatobiliary and Pancreatic Surgery, Trauma and Acute Care Surgery, University of Calgary, Foothills Medical Centre, Calgary, AB, Canada
e-mail: ball.chad@gmail.com

E. Dixon
Hepatobiliary and Pancreatic Surgery, Division of General Surgery, Faculty of Medicine, Foothills Medical Centre, Calgary, AB, Canada

© Springer International Publishing AG 2018
C.G. Ball, E. Dixon (eds.), *Treatment of Ongoing Hemorrhage*,
DOI 10.1007/978-3-319-63495-1_13

these are the gastroepiploic trunk and the first jejunal venous branch (Fig. 13.1). Hemorrhage from these structures can be torrential and unforgiving.

Although portal venous injuries in a retropancreatic location are notoriously difficult to access, human anatomy has provided us with a typically successful maneuver. More specifically, digital pressure from the front of the gland is often adequate to temporarily control venous hemorrhage via simple compression. In cases where this fails, a rapid Kocher maneuver is required to allow concurrent anterior and posterior digital pressure and therefore occlusion of the portal vein and distal SMV itself. This maneuver buys the surgeon time to add a second suction device, call for experienced help, prepare the anesthesiologist for massive blood loss, and have the nursing staff ready all of the vascular instrumentation and suture selections he/she will require. If the hemorrhage appears to be coming from the bottom of the pancreas (i.e., uncinate/head), it is also helpful to rapidly mobilize the right colon to provide improved inferior exposure and eventually control. As with most massive hemorrhage, the importance of an educated assistant who can expose the venous injury (both suctioning of blood and retraction of adjacent organs) cannot be overstated. Excellent help is typically the difference between completing an efficient and smooth repair compared to flailing with massive blood loss and poor direction.

If pressure and packing do not persistently control hemorrhage from the retropancreatic portion of the portal vein moving forward (although this is very unusual), then rapid exposure and subsequent ligation/repair of the vessel may be required. This can be achieved by dividing the neck/body of the pancreas itself (i.e., to allow direct visualization of the vessel). This maneuver is discussed significantly more often in the literature than it is actually performed in the real world. It also carries with it a substantial risk of inadvertently enlarging the venous injury (given near ubiquitous rough dissection in a poorly visualized field). If this maneuver is triggered, however, rapidly place four retraction sutures (3-0 Prolene on MH needles) through the pancreatic neck in a figure-of-eight manner immediately lateral and medial to the portal vein (at both the top and bottom of the gland) (Fig. 13.2). There is significant risk of ligating the hepatic artery at the top, so you must be extremely accurate. This is not the time to flail or lose focus. These four sutures will provide significant retraction from both sides of the pancreatic neck, allowing the surgeon to use high-voltage Bovie electrocautery to transect the pancreas down to the vein quickly. Remember that the vein is not typically dissected off of the back of the pancreas (i.e., like an elective pancreaticoduodenectomy), so you need to slow down as you get closer to the posterior margin of the pancreas. Repairs to the portal or superior mesenteric veins themselves are generally performed with a 5-0 or 6-0 Prolene (once control is obtained with proximal and distal vascular clamps or digital pressure and exposure by an experienced colleague).

In the heat of the battle, venous tributaries from the portal vein can generally be ligated. Furthermore, even the portal vein itself can be ligated in a damage control scenario. Interestingly, these patients display a superior survival when evaluating the literature as a whole compared to portal and superior mesenteric venous repairs. This is not overly surprising and likely reflects the comfort level and rapidity among various surgeons attempting to address these difficult injuries. Another possibility is

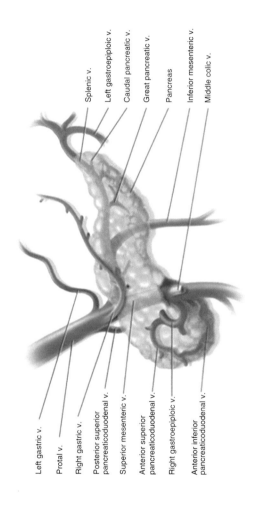

Fig. 13.1 Mesenteric venous anatomy, including the gastroepiploic trunk

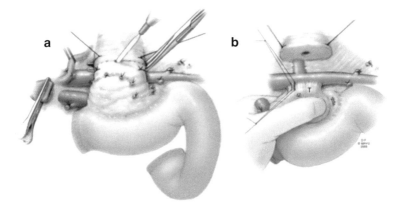

Fig. 13.2 Pancreatic neck traction sutures. (**a**) Distal pancreatic retraction sutures (**b**) Exposed peripancreatic venous confluence

to place a temporary intravascular shunt (TIVS) in continuity for major portal venous injuries. Portal veins are best shunted with a 22–26 French chest tube or large nasogastric feeding tube for small women (please see the Damage Control Chap. 16). Once inserted into the vessel in an in-line manner, the TIVS can be locked into place via either silk ties or double-vessel loops that are tightened/locked with clips. If silk ties are selected (generally more secure for venous structures), it must be remembered that the vessel itself will need to be trimmed back proximal to the silk to ensure there is no ischemia at the time of the reconstruction. This may become a problem for the surgeon in areas where every bit of vessel length is critical (i.e., necessitating a graft at the time of reconstruction).

Ongoing hemorrhage from the splenic vein is much less treacherous than from the portal and superior mesenteric veins. Bleeding to the anatomic left of the portal vein can be solved via a rapid distal pancreatectomy/splenectomy with bulk ligation of the splenic artery and vein. Energy instrumentation and staplers can make this endeavor simple and efficient. More specifically, divide the short gastrics and gastroepiploics, mobilize the transverse and left colon, and finally free the spleen with the energy instrument (LigaSure Impact, Covidien). This instrument even works well under water! A multitude of staplers can then be effectively utilized to divide the pancreatic body concurrent to ligation of the splenic artery and vein. The TX-30 linear stapler (Ethicon) in particular is a workhorse of the elective HPB surgeon and is superb for this indication. Alternatively, in the context of a soft gland, a laparoscopic stapler (with a 60 mm length vascular load) can also be used to divide these structures en masse. The dominant risk is mistaking the hepatic for the proximal splenic artery and dividing it. A quick test clamp of the splenic artery with a large bulldog clamp (to ensure a normal persistent pulse within the porta hepatis) eliminates this potential disaster. Prior to placing either stapler type, however, the surgeon must rapidly dissect around the pancreatic body and place a vessel loop or umbilical tape for complete control of the gland. This is often best done with a single well-educated finger. Remember that the retroperitoneum at this location (i.e., aorta is deep to this site) is generally spared from hemorrhage and easily accessible from the bottom once the transverse colon is mobilized caudally by approximately 1 cm. The splenic vein will remain stuck to the underside of the elevated pancreas, and the splenic artery can be palpated. Although this short series of maneuvers may sound challenging, it becomes much easier when rapidity is in demand. The most extreme damage control maneuver for a splenic venous injury would also remain bulk ligation with a large suture, followed by packing.

While it is beyond the aims of this chapter, the dominant postoperative complications surrounding pancreatic (and duodenal) injuries remain leaks from preceding pancreatoduodenal closures and/or anastomoses. Critically injured patients rarely tolerate the physiologic consequences of uncontrolled leaks. Pancreatic juices are also highly dangerous in the context of a fresh vascular repair, anastomosis, or TIVS. As a result, generous closed suction drainage must be considered to control any potential pancreatic leaks after the ongoing hemorrhage has been stopped. As experienced HPB and trauma surgeons will confirm, intraoperative planning (and therefore procedure selection) for a patient's major postoperative complications is essential.

In summary, massive ongoing hemorrhage associated with pancreatic trauma is typically compressible with a well-educated hand/finger. A detailed knowledge of anatomy and a talented assistant will make the difference between a huge save and a long presentation at morbidity and mortality conference.

Take-Home Points
1. A detailed knowledge of peripancreatic venous anatomy is essential.
2. Most ongoing hemorrhage can be temporized by well-placed finger(s).
3. Damage control maneuvers include both ligation and TIVS.
4. Energy instruments and staplers can be a real lifesaver!
5. Remember the potential pancreatic leak, because it will remember you!

A surgeon operates as good as his assistant permits; so have plenty of assistance, but not many assistants. Augustus C. Bernays

Chapter 14
Genitourinary and Splenic Hemorrhage: We're Important Organs Too!

Stefan W. Leichtle and Kenji Inaba

Case Scenario

A 19-year-old male sustains a single gunshot wound to his left thoracoabdominal area. He is hypotensive and once explored requires both splenectomy and left nephrectomy…

Genitourinary Trauma

Before discussing the evaluation and treatment of patients with suspected or confirmed renal injury, this section will start with concise instructions for an emergent nephrectomy. The authors prefer a lateral approach (described here), but the alternative medial approach will also be discussed and described later in the chapter.

- Position the patient supine, with arms abducted and surgical prep from sternal notch to knees in standard trauma fashion.
- Perform a midline laparotomy incision followed by either packing of all four quadrants in blunt trauma or focused exploration in penetrating trauma.
- Divide the lateral attachments of ascending or descending colon to perform a right or left medial visceral rotation, respectively.
- Open Gerota's fascia laterally and identify kidney and structures of the hilum.
- Control bleeding from the kidney by compressing the hilum manually or with a vascular clamp.

S.W. Leichtle (✉)
Division of Acute Care Surgical Services, Virginia Commonwealth University Medical Center, Richmond, VA, USA
e-mail: stefan.leichtle@vcuhealth.org

K. Inaba
Division of Trauma & Critical Care, LAC+USC Medical Center, Los Angeles, CA, USA

© Springer International Publishing AG 2018
C.G. Ball, E. Dixon (eds.), *Treatment of Ongoing Hemorrhage*,
DOI 10.1007/978-3-319-63495-1_14

- Individually ligate the renal artery, vein, and ureter. The latter should be pursued as distal as possible toward its insertion into the bladder to avoid the development of reflux into the blind-ending ureter. For patients in extremis, mass ligation of the renal hilum is acceptable (via stapler or suture).
- After nephrectomy, avoid nephrotoxic medication and intravenous (IV) contrast. Ensure adequate hydration and monitor urine output and serum creatinine levels.

Background

Though genitourinary (GU) trauma is relatively rare, renal injury is found in 1–5% of trauma patients [1, 2]. Blunt traumas with direct impact to the flank or an acceleration-deceleration mechanism are the most frequent etiologies, but penetrating trauma is a common cause in urban trauma centers. Macroscopic hematuria mandates further evaluation of the kidneys and bladder, while microscopic hematuria in a stable patient does not need to be investigated in the immediate trauma setting. However, a high index of suspicion for GU injuries is necessary as up to one third of patients with renal injuries may present without obvious hematuria [1].

The focused assessment with sonography for trauma (FAST) exam is often negative even in the presence of renal injury due to their retroperitoneal location. In a hemodynamically stable patient, computed tomography (CT) scan of the abdomen and pelvis with intravenous (IV) contrast is the best modality to identify and characterize renal injuries. The revised American Association for the Surgery of Trauma (AAST) classification system from 2011 [3] grades traumatic renal injuries from I to V, with higher grades indicating more severe parenchymal destruction.

Grades I, II, and III describe hematuria or presence of a subcapsular hematoma; perirenal hematoma or a parenchymal laceration of less than 1 cm length; and lacerations through the renal cortex of more than 1 cm in length, respectively. Any injury to the collecting duct system results in classification as grade IV, which also includes vascular injury to the segmental renal vessels. Grade V is reserved for lacerations to or avulsions of the main renal vessels, as well as renal artery or vein thrombosis. The AAST grading system is also clinically relevant, because higher grades correlate with decreased renal salvage rates and increased risk of developing complications.

An isolated renal injury is rarely the cause for hemodynamic instability in a trauma patient, and other sources of hemorrhage need to be ruled out. In any patient undergoing exploratory laparotomy for trauma, zone II of the retroperitoneum containing the kidney should be inspected for the presence of a hematoma (Fig. 14.1). Unless an expanding hematoma or active bleeding is present, Gerota's fascia should not be opened. An intact fascia provides an effective envelope that can tamponade bleeding and prevent urinary leakage. In case Gerota's fascia does need to be opened, a vertical incision should be performed on its lateral aspect to avoid iatrogenic injury to the renal vessels and ureter.

Fig. 14.1 Location of the kidneys in zone II of the retroperitoneum and their relation to renal arteries, veins, and ureters (Reprinted with the permission of Cambridge University Press from [16])

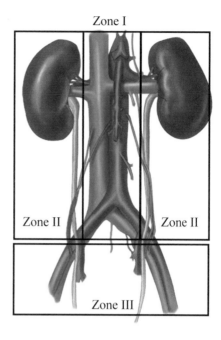

The vast majority of renal injuries (up to 90% in most series) can be successfully managed without operative intervention [3]. In contrast to other solid organ injuries, this is true even for high-grade lacerations. Renal preservation is successful in up to 100% of grade I to III, 80–90% of grade IV, and 5–10% of grade V injuries [3, 4]. Long-term renal function, however, might be diminished in nonoperatively managed grade V injuries and correlates with the amount of devitalized parenchyma [4].

Anatomical Considerations

A brief review of the relevant anatomy is helpful and will facilitate a fast and safe operation. The kidneys are located in zone II of the retroperitoneum. The psoas muscle is adjacent to each kidney medially, and the superior pole of each kidney touches the diaphragm at the level of the eleventh and twelfth rib on the left and right, respectively. The right kidney is located lateral to the duodenum and partially behind the hepatic flexure of the colon. The left kidney lies lateral to the pancreatic tail, inferior to the spleen (connected via splenorenal ligament), and posterior to the splenic flexure of the colon. Each kidney is enveloped by Gerota's fascia.

The renal arteries, originating from the aorta just below the superior mesenteric artery (SMA), provide the blood supply to the kidneys. The other two structures of the renal hilum are the renal vein, located anterior to the artery, and the ureter, which originates from the renal pelvis inferior and posterior to the renal vessels. Each main renal artery splits into several segmental branches that enter the renal hilum. The right renal vein is short (2–4 cm) and drains directly into the inferior vena cava (IVC). The left renal vein is 6–10 cm long and crosses the aorta anteriorly before reaching the IVC. It also receives the left adrenal vein, gonadal vein, and lumbar veins. Therefore, ligation of the left renal vein close to the IVC is possible without incurring venous obstruction and subsequent infarction, while ligation of the right renal vein mandates nephrectomy.

Surgical Technique

Available equipment in the operating room should include a standard laparotomy tray and a Balfour or Bookwalter retractor. A vessel-sealing device such as the LigaSure™ (Medtronic, Minneapolis, MN) can be helpful. The patient is placed supine with both arms abducted, prepped, and draped sterilely from the sternal notch to knees in standard trauma fashion.

A midline laparotomy provides rapid access to the abdominal cavity and good exposure to explore all quadrants. The incision is carried out quickly through the skin and subcutaneous tissues with knife and/or electrocautery. Systematic packing of all four quadrants and evacuation of blood should be performed if the source of hemorrhage is unclear, while a more targeted approach focusing on the right or left retroperitoneum can be chosen if the kidney as a source of hemorrhage is clear from preoperative imaging. As mentioned above, most renal lacerations do not require exploration of the retroperitoneum. In fact, Gerota's fascia should not be opened unless there is a perinephric hematoma that is either expanding or actively bleeding through a defect in the fascia. Before embarking on the exploration of a zone II hematoma, any intra-abdominal bleeding should be addressed first as Gerota's fascia will provide at least temporary tamponade of renal hemorrhage.

Two different approaches to the kidney are possible. The lateral approach is preferred by trauma surgeons due to superior speed and familiarity. It focuses on rapid exposure of the injured kidney with a right or left medial visceral rotation. The medial approach is more often used in elective operations and focuses on proximal vascular control, thus theoretically minimizing blood loss and potentially increasing the chance for organ salvage. As in many trauma situations, the best approach is the one that the operating surgeon is most familiar with.

Lateral Approach

This approach relies on fast, direct access to the injured kidney without prior vascular control. Medial visceral rotation of the right ("Cattell-Braasch maneuver") or left ("modified Mattox maneuver") exposes the kidney (Fig. 14.2). Gerota's fascia is subsequently incised on its lateral aspect and finger dissection is used to rapidly

Fig. 14.2 Left medial visceral rotation to expose the left kidney (Reprinted with the permission of Cambridge University Press from [16])

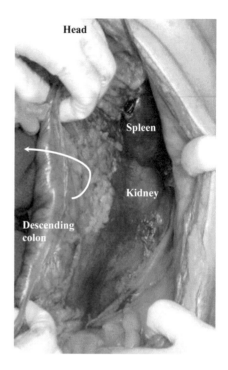

deliver the kidney out of the retroperitoneum and toward the middle. This allows for hemorrhage control via manual compression of the parenchyma and vascular control of the hilum. Vascular control can be achieved by compressing the hilum manually or by application of a non-crushing vascular clamp.

Medial Approach

This approach allows for proximal control of the renal arteries at their origin off the aorta prior to opening Gerota's fascia and exposing the injured kidney. Upward retraction of the transverse colon toward the patient's chest exposes the ligament of Treitz at the base of the transverse mesocolon. Packing of the small bowel toward the right upper quadrant exposes the root of the mesentery and provides access to the aorta in zone I of the retroperitoneum (Fig. 14.1). A longitudinal incision is made in the posterior peritoneum overlying the aorta. The incision is extended cranially up to the point where the left renal vein crosses the aorta (Fig. 14.3). A vessel loop around the vein can help with retraction to expose the posteriorly located left renal artery. The right renal artery is more difficult to access. It lies posterior to the IVC and originates from the posterolateral aspect of the aorta. After obtaining vascular control of the left or right renal artery, the kidney itself can be exposed via left or right medial visceral rotation as described above.

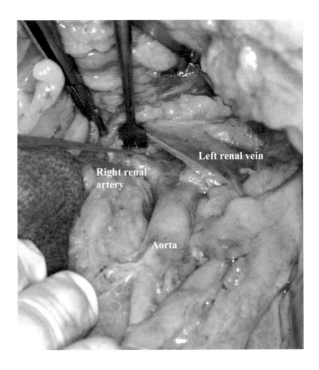

Fig. 14.3 Medial approach to the aorta and control of the right renal artery (with vessel loop) (Reprinted with the permission of Cambridge University Press from [16])

Renal Repair, Partial Nephrectomy, and Nephrectomy

In the hemodynamically unstable, massively injured, or coagulopathic patient, little time should be spent to attempt salvage of a severely damaged kidney. In general, if renal trauma requires operative exploration of the lateral retroperitoneum, a nephrectomy is quite a likely outcome. Nevertheless, in a reasonably stable patient, repair and salvage of the kidney should be considered and attempted.

Renal contusions and subcapsular hematomas, i.e., grade I to III injuries, should be left alone if at all possible. Minor parenchymal hemorrhage can be stopped with manual compression, careful use of electrocautery, argon beam, or suture ligation of bleeding vessels. Once hemostasis has been achieved, devitalized tissue should be debrided and the collecting duct system examined. Any injuries to the latter should be repaired with absorbable, monofilament 4-0 suture to avoid creating a nidus for kidney stone formation. The capsule can be repaired using 2-0 or 3-0 absorbable or nonabsorbable sutures with pledgets (Fig. 14.4).

An omental pedicle or thrombin-soaked Gelfoam® (Pfizer Inc) can be used in situations where extensive tissue loss prohibits primary closure of the capsule (Fig. 14.5).

If severe damage is limited to the superior or inferior pole of the kidney, a partial nephrectomy should be considered. The renal capsule should be dissected off the damaged parenchyma prior to resection, which will facilitate subsequent closure. After transection of the damaged pole, bleeding vessels and injuries to the collecting

Fig. 14.4 Renal capsule repair reinforced with pledgets (Reprinted with the permission of Cambridge University Press from [16])

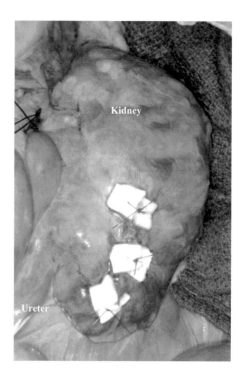

Fig. 14.5 Hemostasis using a Gelfoam® bolster for a deep laceration involving the inferior renal pole (Reprinted with the permission of Cambridge University Press from [16])

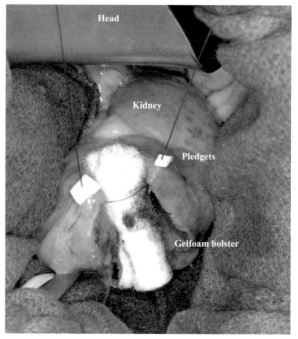

duct system should be repaired with 4-0 absorbable sutures. Additionally, the repair techniques described above including omentum and/or Gelfoam® can be used to reinforce the repair or create a hemostatic bolster. After repair or partial nephrectomy, a closed suction drain should be left in the retroperitoneum.

Traumatic injury to the renal artery in a hemodynamically unstable patient necessitates nephrectomy. In a stable patient with a low associated injury burden, repair of the renal artery can be attempted following general vascular principles, i.e., proximal and distal control with vessel loops or vascular clamps and subsequent repair with 5-0 or 6-0 nonabsorbable monofilament suture. Any nonviable tissue should be debrided and inflow as well as back bleeding assessed. Thrombectomy with a Fogarty catheter might be necessary. Lastly, if injury pattern requires ligation of the renal vein, the side of the injury determines whether the kidney can be saved or not. On the left side, adrenal, gonadal, and lumbar veins provide collateral venous outflow as long as renal vein ligation occurs close to the IVC. Ligation of the right renal vein mandates nephrectomy due to complete venous outflow obstruction.

Topical Energy Application

Hemostatic energy instruments such as the Aquamantys (Medtronic) or Argon Beamer may also be extremely helpful for arresting major (Aquamantys) and/or minor (Aquamantys or Argon Beamer) hemorrhage from the kidney. Although both instruments are easy to use, the Aquamantys is particularly adept at arresting a multitude of types of solid organ lacerations.

Postoperative Management of Renal Trauma

Traditionally, nonoperatively managed high-grade renal injuries (AAST III or higher) underwent mandatory follow-up abdominal CT scan 48–72 h after the injury to detect complications such as renal infarction, pseudoaneurysm, or urinary leakage. However, the incidence of these complications ranges from low to moderate with clinical management rarely changing based on the results of early CT imaging [2]. Therefore, repeat imaging after renal trauma should be guided by clinical concerns or laboratory abnormalities.

After unilateral nephrectomy, serum creatinine is expected to double. As the remaining kidney compensates for the loss of the other, serum creatinine should decline over time to levels at or slightly above baseline. To avoid damage to the single remaining kidney, nephrotoxic medications (e.g., nonsteroidal anti-inflammatory drugs, certain antibiotics) and IV contrast must be avoided. The patient should undergo adequate resuscitation and hydration and strict urine output monitoring. Hypoperfusion secondary to hypotensive episodes should be avoided. Urinary leakage is a more common complication and might require treatment via ureteral stenting or percutaneous nephrostomy. Any postoperative urinoma should be drained percutaneously. The late development of renovascular hypotension is exceedingly rare.

Pitfalls and Complications

Missed Injury to the Collecting Duct System

Urinary leakage and urinoma formation can be the consequences of missed injuries to the renal calices and/or collecting duct system. If stability of the patient allows, intraoperative retrograde injection of methylene blue through a 22 g butterfly needle into the ureter can demonstrate subtle injuries to the collecting duct system. Repair should be watertight with an absorbable 4-0 monofilament suture. A drain can help detect urinary leakage early and prevent spillage of urine into the peritoneal cavity after repair. Closed-suction drains should be placed after all renal repairs and partial nephrectomies.

Suturing of Renal Parenchyma and Capsule

The renal parenchyma does not hold sutures well, and preservation of the capsule during parenchymal debridement or transection can facilitate subsequent repair and closure tremendously. Sutures through the capsule can be reinforced using pledgets, Gelfoam, or omentum. The latter two can also be used to cover larger areas of parenchymal or capsular defects.

Effect of Urinary Leakage on Other Abdominal Injuries

While postoperative urinary leakage does not appear to adversely affect long-term renal function [4], it compromises wound healing and may increase the risk for dehiscence of nearby bowel anastomoses. Therefore, closed-suction drains should always be placed after repair or partial resection of the kidney. The omentum, fascia, or muscle can be used to separate the damaged kidney from the peritoneal cavity.

The Spleen

Before discussing the evaluation and treatment of patients with suspected or confirmed splenic injury, this chapter will start with step-by-step instructions for an emergent splenectomy:

- Position the patient supine with arms abducted, and surgical prep from the sternal notch to knees in standard trauma fashion.

- Perform a midline laparotomy incision followed by packing of all four quadrants in blunt trauma or focused exploration of the left upper quadrant in penetrating trauma to the spleen.
- Mobilize the spleen toward the middle by packing three to four laparotomy pads behind the spleen over your non-dominant hand.
- Divide the avascular splenic attachments to the kidney, colon, and diaphragm (splenorenal, splenocolic, and phrenosplenic ligament) using blunt or sharp dissection.
- Control the splenic hilum manually or with a non-crushing clamp to arrest hemorrhage.
- Divide the gastrosplenic ligament, which contains the short gastric vessels using clamp-and-tie technique or a vessel-sealing device such as the LigaSure™. Stay close to the spleen to avoid injury to the stomach.
- Individually ligate the splenic artery and vein with suture ligatures. Stay close to the spleen to avoid damage to the pancreatic tail. If there is any concern for injury to the distal pancreas, leave a closed-suction drain in the lesser sac.
- After splenectomy, assess the most common sites of postoperative bleeding for hemostasis: the ligated splenic hilum and the short gastric vessels.
- Administer vaccines against encapsulated bacteria (meningococcus, pneumococcus, *H. influenzae*) prior to hospital discharge for an emergent splenectomy.

Background

Splenic injury most often occurs through direct blunt impact to the left flank. It should be also be suspected if there is severe left upper quadrant pain and an abdominal seatbelt sign and if left lower rib fractures are present. In penetrating trauma, any injury to the left thoracoabdominal area should raise concern for splenic trauma. The FAST exam is an excellent tool to detect free abdominal fluid and is often positive in the left upper quadrant in the setting of splenic injury. In a hemodynamically stable patient, a positive FAST exam should be followed by a CT scan of the abdomen and pelvis with IV contrast as isolated solid organ injuries can frequently be managed nonoperatively. A positive FAST exam in a hemodynamically unstable patient (hypotension, tachycardia, or narrow pulse pressure) or peritonitis on physical exam should lead to immediate operative intervention.

The majority of splenic injuries can be managed nonoperatively. Though there is a lack of data from randomized controlled trials, numerous retrospective and prospective observational studies reported success rates of up to 90% [5–8] for nonoperative management (NOM) of isolated, low- to moderate-grade splenic injuries. The average success rate including all severities of injury is about 70% in adult patients and even higher in pediatric trauma. The contribution of angiographic embolization to the success rate of NOM is controversial, and data is conflicting [5, 7]. Moderate- to high-grade splenic injuries increase the risk for the development of pseudoaneurysms, in which case angioembolization is clearly indicated to prevent late hemorrhage. In general, splenic injuries of grade III or higher and those with active extravasation on abdominal CT should at least be referred for evaluation by interventional radiology unless other indications for splenectomy are present.

The AAST classifies splenic injuries from grade I to V based on imaging and/or intraoperative findings [9]. Success rates of nonoperative management and approaches to treatment correlate with these grades to some degree [10], although the reliability of imaging findings in predicting outcomes has been questioned [11]. Grades I and II describe minor lacerations and subcapsular hematomas that can often be observed. Grade III injuries, comprising larger subcapsular hematomas, lacerations of more than 3 cm length, and ruptured parenchymal hematomas, are less likely to stop bleeding without intervention. Some advocate for routine angio-embolization of splenic injuries with active extravasation; others reserve it for patients with pseudoaneurysms or signs of persistent low-grade bleeding. Nonoperative management of patients with grade IV lacerations is sometimes successful. This course of action mandates admission to the intensive care unit (ICU), close monitoring, and evaluation for angiographic embolization. If operative intervention is required, consideration can be given to splenic repair and preservation, particularly in younger patients with isolated splenic injury. Patients with a shattered spleen or injury to the splenic hilum (grade V) are at high risk for exsanguination and unlikely to avoid a splenectomy. Major trauma organizations including the Western Trauma Association (WTA) [12] and Eastern Association for the Surgery of Trauma (EAST) [13] have developed algorithms and guidelines for the management of splenic injuries based on the best available current evidence.

It is critical to recognize when nonoperative treatment of splenic injury needs to be abandoned. Persistent right upper quadrant pain, decreasing hemoglobin levels, and the need for multiple blood transfusions (the exact number is controversial) should prompt critical reevaluation of the nonoperative strategy. Hemodynamic instability, worsening abdominal pain, the development of peritonitis, and associated head injury are indications for immediate operative intervention.

Anatomical Considerations

A brief review of the relevant anatomy is helpful and will facilitate a fast and safe operation. The spleen is located deep in the left upper quadrant, covered by the ninth to eleventh ribs (Fig. 14.6). It is in close proximity to the diaphragm, stomach, pancreatic tail, kidney, and colon. Four ligamentous attachments connect the spleen to its adjacent structures: phrenosplenic, splenorenal, splenocolic, and gastrosplenic ligament. The length of these ligaments and the proximity of the splenic hilum to the pancreatic tail are variable and have considerable influence on the degree of difficulty mobilizing and resecting the spleen. Except for the highly vascular gastro-splenic ligament, which contains the short gastric vessels, all splenic ligaments can be divided bluntly if needed, though sharp division is ideal. Frequently, a large perisplenic hematoma has already done much of the dissection for the surgeon.

Fig. 14.6 Location of the spleen in the left upper quadrant (Reprinted with the permission of Cambridge University Press from [16])

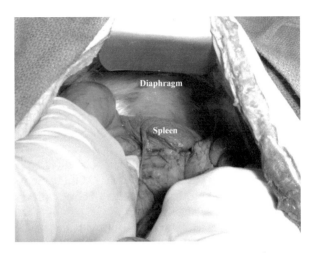

The splenic hilum consists of splenic artery and vein. The former originates from the celiac trunk, courses superiorly along the edge of the pancreas, and splits up into a superior and inferior pole artery at the hilum. There is a variable branch pattern with two thirds of patients having multiple vessels that split up as far as 5–10 cm away from the spleen and one third of patients having two main vessels branching close to the spleen. The splenic vein lies posterior and inferior to the artery. It receives the inferior mesenteric vein (IMV) and eventually forms the portal vein when joined by the superior mesenteric vein (SMV).

Surgical Technique

Available equipment in the operating room should include a standard laparotomy tray, Balfour or Bookwalter retractors, as well as pledgets and mesh if splenic salvage is to be attempted. A vessel-sealing device such as the LigaSure™ can be helpful. The patient is placed supine with both arms abducted, prepped from the sternal notch to knees in standard trauma fashion.

A midline laparotomy provides rapid access to the abdominal cavity and good exposure to explore all quadrants. The midline laparotomy incision is carried out quickly through the skin and subcutaneous tissues with knife and/or electrocautery. Systematic packing of all four quadrants and evacuation of blood should be performed if the source of hemorrhage is unclear, while a more targeted approach focusing on the left upper quadrant can be chosen if the spleen has been identified as source of hemorrhage due to mechanism or on preoperative imaging. A handheld Richardson retractor can provide adequate exposure for initial packing of the left upper quadrant, but a Bookwalter retractor is helpful for optimal exposure.

Mobilization of the spleen toward the midline is a crucial maneuver to assess the extent of damage to the spleen and perform repairs and partial resections or a rapid

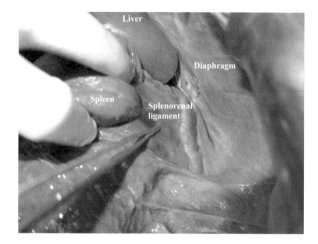

Fig. 14.7 The splenorenal ligament is one of the three nonvascular attachments of the spleen (in addition to phrenosplenic and splenocolic ligaments) (Reprinted with the permission of Cambridge University Press from [16])

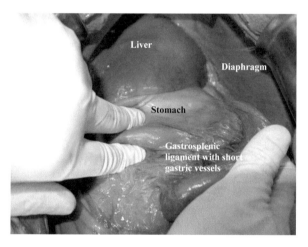

Fig. 14.8 The gastrosplenic ligament is of variable length and contains the short gastric vessels (Reprinted with the permission of Cambridge University Press from [16])

splenectomy. Packing in the left upper quadrant aims to achieve temporary arrest of hemorrhage and improves exposure by bringing the spleen toward the middle. The surgeon's non-dominant hand slides over the spleen and gently pulls the organ in inferomedial direction. With the dominant hand, three to four laparotomy pads are subsequently packed behind the spleen until it has been mobilized well toward the midline. In high-grade injuries, the large perisplenic hematoma has often done most of the dissection and facilitates mobilization of the organ. If not, the phrenosplenic, splenorenal (Fig. 14.7), and splenocolic ligaments need to be divided bluntly or sharply to fully bring the spleen to the midline. Traction on the latter is often the cause for capsular tears during colectomies during mobilization of the splenic flexure of the colon. When dividing the splenocolic ligament, injury to the colon in close proximity needs to be avoided.

The fourth ligament of the spleen, the gastrosplenic ligament (Fig. 14.8), contains the short gastric vessels and as such is a highly vascular structure requiring division via clamp-and-tie technique. Alternatively, this can be achieved more rapidly with a vessel-sealing device. The short gastric vessels should be divided as close to the spleen as possible to avoid injury to or devascularization of the greater curvature of the stomach.

With the spleen in midline, the splenic hilum can be clamped manually or with a non-crushing clamp. This immediately arrests hemorrhage and allows for inspection of the spleen. At this point, several options exist:

- Splenectomy
- Partial splenectomy
- Splenorrhaphy
- Topical hemostasis

The decision on whether to salvage or take the spleen needs to be made weighing the risks and benefits of either approach in the individual trauma patient. Associated traumatic brain injuries, presence of coagulopathy and hypothermia, or substantial splenic parenchymal destruction or devascularization are indications for splenectomy. Young age, hemodynamic stability, and a low-grade or localized splenic injury on the other hand make splenic preservation a viable option. Lastly, personal comfort and experience as well as postoperative care (ICU in level I trauma center vs. limited resources in a combat zone) should be taken into consideration.

Splenectomy

With the spleen mobilized toward the midline and all four ligaments divided, only the splenic hilum remains to be transected. Individual ligation of the splenic artery and vein are preferred. This technique minimizes the risk for late development of an arteriovenous fistula and damage to the pancreatic tail. Double ligation of the splenic vessels with two 3-0 silk suture ligatures provides optimal safety. In damage control situations when splenectomy has to be performed as quickly as possible, stapling across the hilum with a GIA™ stapler or use of a vessel-sealing device allows for rapid splenectomy.

No matter which technique is used to divide the splenic hilum, it is crucial to stay as close to the spleen as possible to avoid inadvertent injury to the distal pancreas. If there is any concern for pancreatic injury, a closed-suction drain should be left in the lesser sac. If an injury is obvious, or if limited exposure requires the pancreatic tail to be taken, a TA™ stapler should be used to transect the pancreatic tail. In these cases, a closed-suction drain should be left in place as well (Fig. 14.9). After removal of the spleen, it is important to assess for good hemostasis. Common bleeding sites are near the tail of pancreas and at the greater gastric curvature at the location of the short gastric vessels. A useful technique is to insert a rolled laparotomy pad deep into the left upper quadrant and to slowly roll it back toward the surgeon while examining all surfaces for signs of bleeding.

Fig. 14.9 Splenectomy
with distal pancreatectomy
using a TA stapler
(Reprinted with the
permission of Cambridge
University Press from [16])

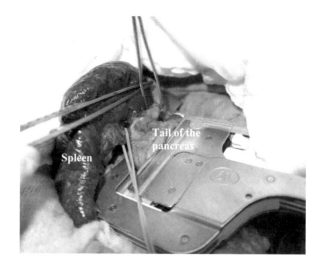

Partial Splenectomy

Partial splenectomy will rarely be a viable option but can be considered if there is isolated injury to the upper or lower pole in a hemodynamically stable patient. The blood supply to the spleen is segmental, and therefore, a part of spleen can be safely removed. Ideally, the individual vessels in the hilar area that supply the pole to be resected should be found and ligated first, before opening the splenic capsule. There are several options for dissection of the parenchyma itself, including opening of the capsule with electrocautery followed by finger dissection of the parenchyma and ligation of individual vessels with 3-0 or 4-0 silk, firing the TA™ stapler across the spleen, or using a vessel-sealing device to cut across the splenic parenchyma. In case of persistent oozing from the cut edge, horizontal mattress sutures and pledgets can be used for reinforcement (Fig. 14.10). Alternatively, an omental pedicle can be wrapped around the spleen by creating a flap of gastrocolic omentum that remains partially connected to the gastroepiploic arcade.

Splenorrhaphy

Splenorrhaphy can be considered if the splenic injury is not amenable to resection of an individual pole but if there is limited parenchymal damage in an otherwise hemodynamically stable patient without severe injury burden. Again, prolonged attempts to salvage the spleen should not be undertaken at the cost of compromising the patient's overall outcome. Excellent exposure and mobilization toward the midline (as described above) are crucial for a successful splenorrhaphy. Capsular tears and areas of bleeding can be repaired with a size 0 chromic suture with a blunt needle ("liver needle") in figure-of-eight or horizontal mattress fashion. This works well if the capsule is still intact; if not, pledgets can be used to reinforce the suture

Fig. 14.10 Reinforcement of the cut splenic edge with horizontal mattress sutures using pledgets and chromic suture with a blunt needle (Reprinted with the permission of Cambridge University Press from [16])

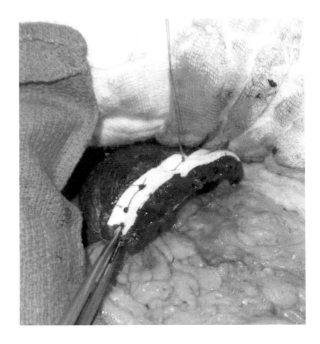

line (Fig. 14.10). Importantly, deep bleeding requires exploration and ligation of the offending vessel. If the capsule is just closed over such an injury, development of an intraparenchymal hematoma or pseudoaneurysm with delayed rupture can be the serious consequences.

Alternatively, the entire spleen can be wrapped in a Vicryl mesh or a commercially available bag. Data on the effectiveness of such techniques is very limited. The key to these maneuvers again is complete mobilization of the spleen. The mesh wrap can be supplemented with topical hemostatic. It needs to be emphasized again that time-consuming maneuvers to repair the spleen should not be performed at the cost of a prolonged stay in the operating room with a severely injured patient.

Topical Hemostatic

Techniques for topical hemostasis include the use of clotting matrices such as Surgicel® (Ethicon) or Gelfoam®/thrombin and coagulation devices including electrocautery and argon beam. When attempting topical hemostasis, full mobilization of the spleen with transection of all ligaments might not be necessary as long as adequate exposure can be achieved.

In the severely injured polytrauma patient whose presentation is often complicated by coagulopathy and hypothermia, it is best to choose any method that is reasonably fast and simple.

Topical Energy Application

Hemostatic energy instruments such as the Aquamantys (Medtronic) or Argon Beamer may also be extremely helpful for arresting major (Aquamantys) and/or minor (Aquamantys or Argon Beamer) hemorrhage from the spleen. Although both instruments are easy to use, the Aquamantys is particularly adept at arresting a multitude of types of solid organ lacerations.

Pitfalls and Complications

Diaphragmatic Injury

In patients with penetrating splenic trauma, there is a high risk of concomitant diaphragmatic injury. The combination of left-sided hemothorax and splenic injury is pathognomonic of diaphragmatic laceration. Therefore, the diaphragm should always be examined intraoperatively. If a patient successfully undergoes nonoperative management of a splenic injury, diagnostic laparoscopy should be offered after a period of observation and after other injuries have been ruled out (usually 24–48 h). If a diaphragmatic injury is found, conversion to a laparotomy might be necessary depending on the surgeon's laparoscopy skills.

In an open procedure, long Allis clamps are excellent tools to bring the diaphragmatic tear into view, grasp, and approximate the edges to close the defect. Closure should be performed with a large, nonabsorbable suture such as Prolene® (Ethicon). In case of associated bowel injury, the chest should be washed out through the diaphragm before closure. After repair of any diaphragmatic injury, an ipsilateral 28 Fr chest tube should be placed.

Injuries during Dissection

After mobilization of the spleen, the short gastric vessels should be transected as close to the spleen as possible to avoid direct or thermal (when using a vessel-sealing device) injury to the stomach. If there is any concern for gastric injury, affected areas along the greater gastric curvature should be reinforced with Lembert sutures.

Ligation of the splenic vessels and transection of the splenic hilum should be performed as close to the spleen as possible to avoid injury to the pancreatic tail. The risk for this complication is higher when a stapling or energy device is used as opposed to clamp-and-tie technique for the individual vessels. A drain should be left in the lesser sac if there is any concern for this complication, or a distal pancreatectomy should be performed if injury is obvious.

Persistent Hemorrhage

The most common sites of persistent bleeding after splenectomy are near the tail of the pancreas and along the greater gastric curvature where the short gastric vessels insert. These sites should be closely examined after splenectomy. A rolled laparotomy pad, inserted deep into the left upper quadrant and slowly rolled back toward the surgeon, is a helpful technique. Bleeding from these areas requires surgical hemostasis and needs to be differentiated from the diffuse hemorrhage seen in the coagulopathic trauma patient.

Local and Systemic Complications

Complications after splenectomy can be divided into local and systemic complications. The former include bleeding, abscess formation, pancreatic leak, (reactive) pleural effusion, gastric injury, and gastroparesis. Many can be avoided by careful dissection and meticulous operative technique. A pancreatic leak can often be managed nonoperatively if a drain has been left in place during the index operation.

Systemic complications include the rare but very serious overwhelming postsplenectomy infection (OPSI) from encapsulated organisms: *Streptococcus pneumoniae*, *Neisseria meningitidis*, and *Haemophilus influenzae*. All patients should be immunized after splenectomy, though the protective effect of vaccines has been debated [14]. In the trauma population with often inconsistent follow-up, the vaccines should be administered prior to the patient leaving the hospital. In addition to OPSI, patients appear to be at higher risk for infections in general in the postoperative period [15].

Take-Home Points
1. The kidneys are the most commonly injured organs of the genitourinary tract with potential for significant blood loss.
2. In contrast to splenic injuries, nonoperative management of high-grade renal lacerations is frequently successful and generally preferred.
3. Intraoperatively, high-grade renal lacerations can present as zone II retroperitoneal hematoma and should only be explored in select circumstances.
4. Urinary leakage due to genitourinary trauma compromises wound healing and increases the risk for dehiscence of nearby bowel anastomoses. Closed-suction drains mitigate this risk and should always be placed after repair or partial resection of the kidney.
5. The spleen is the most commonly injured organ in blunt trauma.
6. Splenic injuries can be managed nonoperatively with and without angiographic embolization and operatively, which includes splenectomy and techniques for splenic salvage.
7. Hemodynamic instability, peritonitis, and associated intracranial hemorrhage are absolute indications for splenectomy.
8. In nonoperatively managed high-grade splenic injuries, follow-up should include repeat imaging to rule out the formation of pseudoaneurysms.

   You have to ligate the artery if the tip of the diathermy fits into its end. Mosche Schein

References

1. Morey AF, Brandes S, Dugi DD, Armstrong JH, Breyer BN, Broghammer JA, Erickson BA, Holzbeierlein J, Hudak SJ, Pruitt JH, Reston JT, Santucci RA, Smith TG, Wessells H, American Urological A. Urotrauma: AUA guideline. J Urol. 2014;192(2):327–35. doi:10.1016/j.juro.2014.05.004.

2. Bukur M, Inaba K, Barmparas G, Paquet C, Best C, Lam L, Plurad D, Demetriades D. Routine follow-up imaging of kidney injuries may not be justified. J Trauma. 2011;70(5):1229–33. doi:10.1097/TA.0b013e3181e5bb8e.

3. Buckley JC, McAninch JW. Revision of current American Association for the Surgery of Trauma renal injury grading system. J Trauma. 2011;70(1):35–7. doi:10.1097/TA.0b013e318207ad5a.

4. Fiard G, Rambeaud JJ, Descotes JL, Boillot B, Terrier N, Thuillier C, Chodez M, Skowron O, Berod AA, Arnoux V, Long JA. Long-term renal function assessment with dimercapto-succinic acid scintigraphy after conservative treatment of major renal trauma. J Urol. 2012;187(4):1306–9. doi:10.1016/j.juro.2011.11.103.

5. Harbrecht BG, Ko SH, Watson GA, Forsythe RM, Rosengart MR, Peitzman AB. Angiography for blunt splenic trauma does not improve the success rate of nonoperative management. J Trauma. 2007;63(1):44–9. doi:10.1097/TA.0b013e3180686531.

6. Plurad DS, Green DJ, Inaba K, Benfield R, Lam L, Putty B, Demetriades D. Blunt assault is associated with failure of nonoperative management of the spleen independent of organ injury grade and despite lower overall injury severity. J Trauma. 2009;66(3):630–5. doi:10.1097/TA.0b013e3181991aed.

7. Rajani RR, Claridge JA, Yowler CJ, Patrick P, Wiant A, Summers JI, McDonald AA, Como JJ, Malangoni MA. Improved outcome of adult blunt splenic injury: a cohort analysis. Surgery. 2006;140(4):625–631.; discussion 631-622. doi:10.1016/j.surg.2006.07.005.

8. Weinberg JA, Magnotti LJ, Croce MA, Edwards NM, Fabian TC. The utility of serial computed tomography imaging of blunt splenic injury: still worth a second look? J Trauma. 2007;62(5):1143–1147.; discussion 1147-1148. doi:10.1097/TA.0b013e318047b7c2.

9. Moore EE, Cogbill TH, Jurkovich GJ, Shackford SR, Malangoni MA, Champion HR. Organ injury scaling: spleen and liver (1994 revision). J Trauma. 1995;38(3):323–4.

10. Velmahos GC, Zacharias N, Emhoff TA, Feeney JM, Hurst JM, Crookes BA, Harrington DT, Gregg SC, Brotman S, Burke PA, Davis KA, Gupta R, Winchell RJ, Desjardins S, Alouidor R, Gross RI, Rosenblatt MS, Schulz JT, Chang Y. Management of the most severely injured spleen: a multicenter study of the research consortium of New England centers for trauma (ReCONECT). Arch Surg. 2010;145(5):456–60. doi:10.1001/archsurg.2010.58.

11. Cohn SM, Arango JI, Myers JG, Lopez PP, Jonas RB, Waite LL, Corneille MG, Stewart RM, Dent DL. Computed tomography grading systems poorly predict the need for intervention after spleen and liver injuries. Am Surg. 2009;75(2):133–9.

12. Moore FA, Davis JW, Moore EE Jr, Cocanour CS, West MA, McIntyre RC Jr. Western trauma association (WTA) critical decisions in trauma: management of adult blunt splenic trauma. J Trauma. 2008;65(5):1007–11. doi:10.1097/TA.0b013e31818a93bf.

13. Stassen NA, Bhullar I, Cheng JD, Crandall ML, Friese RS, Guillamondegui OD, Jawa RS, Maung AA, Rohs TJ Jr, Sangosanya A, Schuster KM, Seamon MJ, Tchorz KM, Zarzuar BL, Kerwin AJ, Eastern Association for the Surgery of T. Selective nonoperative management of blunt splenic injury: an eastern Association for the Surgery of trauma practice management guideline. J Trauma Acute Care Surg. 2012;73(5 Suppl 4):S294–300. doi:10.1097/TA.0b013e3182702afc.

14. Edgren G, Almqvist R, Hartman M, Utter GH. Splenectomy and the risk of sepsis: a population-based cohort study. Ann Surg. 2014;260(6):1081–7. doi:10.1097/SLA.0000000000000439.

15. Demetriades D, Scalea TM, Degiannis E, Barmparas G, Konstantinidis A, Massahis J, Inaba K. Blunt splenic trauma: splenectomy increases early infectious complications: a prospective multicenter study. J Trauma Acute Care Surg. 2012;72(1):229–34. doi:10.1097/TA.0b013e31823fe0b6.

16. Demetriades D, Inaba K, Velmahos G. Atlas of surgical techniques in trauma. Cambridge: Cambridge University Press; 2015.

Chapter 15
Pelvic Trauma Hemorrhage: How Do We Stop Bleeding in that Space?

Clay Cothren Burlew, Charles Fox, and Ernest E. Moore

Case Scenario

A 64-year-old woman is struck by a motor vehicle. She arrives in extremis and has bilateral open femur fractures and a massive pelvic fracture. Her extended FAST examination does not identify any fluid within her peritoneal cavity.

The vast majority of patients delivered to the emergency department (ED) with a pelvic fracture are hemodynamically stable. But the 5–10% of patients with pelvic fractures arriving in hemorrhagic shock represent a unique challenge. A recent multicenter trial of these patients from 11 level 1 trauma centers from the American Association for the Surgery of Trauma (AAST) reported an alarming mortality of 32% [1]. Previous reviews had suggested that uncontrolled bleeding is the predominant course of death in patients succumbing to major pelvic fractures. The purpose of this overview is to provide a contemporary management approach to life-threatening hemorrhage associated with unstable pelvic fractures. The focus is rapid hemorrhage control emphasizing the relatively new concept of resuscitative endovascular aortic balloon occlusion (REBOA) and peritoneal pelvic packing (PPP) in combination with the accepted standards of ED pelvic binding [2] and goal-directed hemostasis with early blood components [3]. At the same time, it is important to recognize that due to the tremendous energy transfer required to generate an unstable pelvic fracture, many of the patients will sustain concomitant life-threatening injuries. In a recent review of patients with major pelvic fractures, 20% had thoracic trauma, 17% had head injury, 8% had significant liver or spleen trauma, and 8% had >2 long bone fracture [4]. In addition, there may be bladder, urethral, rectal, vaginal, external iliac arterial, and lumbosacral nerve injuries that necessitate early recognition [4].

C.C. Burlew, MD (✉) • C. Fox, MD • E.E. Moore, MD
Department of Surgery, Denver Health Medical Center and University of Colorado
School of Medicine, Denver, CO, USA
e-mail: clay.cothren@dhha.org

C.G. Ball, E. Dixon (eds.), *Treatment of Ongoing Hemorrhage*,
DOI 10.1007/978-3-319-63495-1_15

Initial Assessment and Management

While the basic principles of ATLS apply to all seriously injured patients, the ABCs may not follow this priority in the hemodynamically unstable patient at risk for a major pelvic fracture. This high-risk group includes pedestrians or bicyclists struck by cars, high-speed lateral impact motor vehicle crashes (MVC), and falls >25 ft. In this scenario, if such a patient arrives in hemorrhagic shock (SBP <90 mmHg), a pelvic binder or sheep wrapping of the pelvis should be done immediately without an effort to confirm unstable pelvic fractures by physical exam or radiograph (Fig. 15.1). As red blood cells (RBC) and plasma are being infused, a right common femoral artery (RCFA) catheter should be inserted immediately to enable placement of a REBOA catheter (Prytime, Denver). A viscoelastic hemostatic assay (TEG or ROTEM), arterial blood gas (ABG), and hemoglobin measurement should be obtained for the RCFA line. At this time, the results of an extended FAST should be

Denver Health Unstable Pelvic Fracture Management

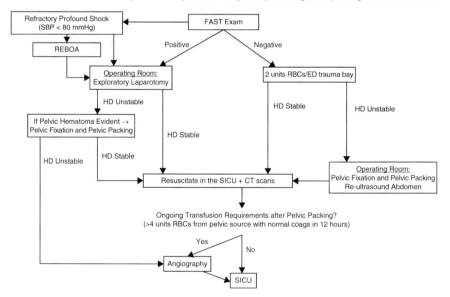

Fig. 15.1 Denver Health Medical Center (DHMC) algorithm for the management of hemodynamically unstable patients with mechanically unstable pelvic fractures (*ATLS* Advanced Trauma Life Support, *CXR* chest radiograph, *FAST* focused abdominal sonographic examination for trauma, *ED* emergency department, *REBOA* resuscitative endovascular balloon occlusion of the aorta, *OR* operating room)

available to exclude a hemopneumothorax that warrants a chest tube and identify hemoperitoneum. If patients SBP remains <80 mmHg, a REBOA should be inflated in zone III before the patient is paralyzed for endotracheal intubation [5].

Resuscitative Endovascular Balloon Occlusion

Currently, there is mixed opinion as to the sequence of therapies and optimal timing of adjunctive maneuvers while transfusing patients presenting in refractory shock with a severe pelvic fracture. Arguably the most significant development in modern vascular surgery is the emergence of endovascular techniques for managing vascular disease, and these techniques are now being extended to traumatic injuries. Although initially applied to injuries for which open repair was highly morbid (thoracic aorta) or provided limited exposure (distal carotid, subclavian artery), endovascular techniques for temporizing acute control of hemorrhage or as definitive management can be applied to a wide array of arterial injury patterns [6–9]. A national analysis demonstrated a 27-fold increase in the use of endovascular therapy, and this was associated with a decrease in morbidity, hospital stay, and mortality [10]. Technical success of these procedures is 90–100% and provides a definitive, minimally invasive treatment option [11]. Resuscitative endovascular balloon occlusion of the aorta (REBOA) has recently emerged as a viable adjunct in the management of patients with non-compressible torso hemorrhage (NCTH) [6, 7]. This intervention is less invasive and may effectively increase central blood pressure (cardiac and cerebral perfusion) and control active pelvic bleeding, potentially obviating the need for resuscitative thoracotomy.

Placement of the REBOA catheter requires femoral arterial (open or percutaneous) access to insert a balloon into the aorta with or without a supporting wire; radiologic imaging is used to confirm proper placement. Enthusiasm for this technique has prompted a reappraisal of aortic balloon occlusion introduced nearly six decades ago during the Korean War. Based on several animal models and an increased number of recent publications, many level I trauma centers in the United States have now opted to use REBOA in patients with refractory hypotension from pelvic hemorrhage.

It appears that REBOA deployed in zone III (Fig. 15.2) may prove to be the optimal means of immediate hemorrhage control in the patient with pelvic fractures in hemorrhagic shock [12]. Transfer of patients to the interventional radiology suite for angioembolization is only appropriate when other sources of major hemorrhage have been excluded, as ongoing hemorrhage in an uncontrolled environment can be disastrous. Moreover, the arterial catheter allows for immediate hemodynamic monitoring and performance of arteriography in the operating room (OR) and eliminates the need for transport to interventional radiology.

Immediate percutaneous femoral arterial cannulation with a 7 French Pinnacle Precision Access System (Terumo Medical, Elkton, MD) is performed on patients

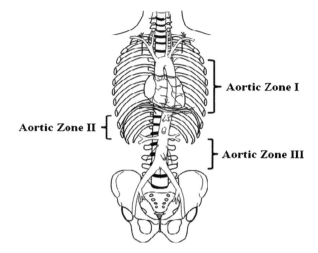

Fig. 15.2 Aortic zones related to REBOA. Zone I extends from the origin of the left subclavian artery to the celiac artery and is a potential zone of occlusion. Zone II extends from the celiac artery to the lowest renal artery and is a no-occlusion zone. Zone III exists from the lowest renal artery to the aortic bifurcation (Reproduced from Stannard et al. [7])

in severe shock with either ultrasound guidance or manual palpation of the femoral artery. Partial responders with systolic blood pressure less than 80 mmHg are treated by placement of the REBOA catheter through the femoral artery sheath. Prepare the device by connecting the monitoring system, flushing the catheter, and removing air from the balloon. A mixture of saline and contrast should be drawn up in a 20 cc syringe for balloon inflation and opacification by digital radiograph (Fig. 15.3). The insertion length of the ER-REBOA™ Catheter is based upon the groin to umbilicus distance for zone III (just above the aortic bifurcation) occlusion. This should be measured externally with the bottom of the balloon located at the umbilicus. One should document the intended location of catheter delivery, which is essential for confirming placement at the intended location. Insert the peel away into the hemostatic valve of the sheath and advance the ER-REBOA™ Catheter under sterile conditions to the appropriate insertion length through the sheath (noted by the external length marks on the catheter shaft). Slide the peel away to the back end of the catheter. Obtain and document pre-inflation vital signs. Flush arterial monitoring port with saline, and inflate ER-REBOA™ balloon using the mixture of saline and contrast. Maximum balloon inflation is 26 mL, but typical volumes used to occlude the aorta are less than 15 mL. Following balloon inflation, vital signs, insertion length, and time of inflation for the catheter are documented. Portable radiography or fluoroscopy is used to confirm the location of the ER-REBOA™ balloon. The femoral sheath and REBOA catheter should be secured prior to patient transport (Fig. 15.3b). Based upon hemodynamic stability, the patient is quickly transferred to the CT scanner or the OR for pelvic packing and external fixation [13]. The REBOA balloon is usually quickly deflated with a goal of less than 3 h of occlusion time.

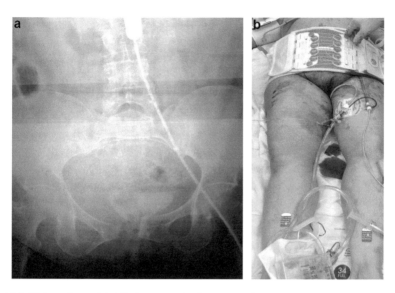

Fig. 15.3 Plain radiograph in ED demonstrating REBOA balloon inflated in REBOA zone III (**a**). The REBOA catheter should be externally secured to the patient prior to transport (**b**)

Pelvic arteriography can easily be performed in the OR using portable fluoroscopy along with other necessary procedures avoiding the additional transportation to a radiology suite.

ED Triage Decision-Making

Assuming the patient has now undergone emergent endotracheal intubation, the anticipated injury pattern and response to the REBOA are important in deciding the next step. As mentioned above, many of these patients harbor additional life-threatening injuries. Thus, if the patient has a robust, sustained response to the REBOA (SBP > 120 mmHg), optimally, a rapid CT scan of the head, cervical spine, chest, abdomen, and pelvis should be considered on the way to the OR. Conversely, if the patient is hemodynamically unstable, they should be taken promptly to the OR for preperitoneal pelvic packing (PPP), external skeletal fixation of the pelvis, and an assessment for the need for a laparotomy.

Preperitoneal Pelvic Packing

Control of pelvic hemorrhage in patients with unstable pelvic fractures can be accomplished with preperitoneal pelvic packing (PPP). Originally described in Europe [14, 15], the technique was modified to directly pack the pelvic space through a preperitoneal approach [16]. Because 85% of pelvic fracture-related bleeding is venous or bony in origin, hemorrhage can be tamponaded within the retroperitoneal space. The combination of pelvic fracture stabilization via external fixation and tamponade of venous bleeding via PPP addresses the two major sources of bleeding. Additionally, the overall potential pelvic space can be reduced by closing down the pelvic volume with surgical stabilization and by filling the pelvic space with packing.

The technique of PPP can be accomplished in under 10 min. A 6–8 cm suprapubic incision is made and the midline fascia is divided. Care is taken not to injure the bladder, which lies directly beneath the incision. The pelvic hematoma, which typically dissects the space, is encountered upon dividing the posterior fascia or with blunt dissection along the posterior aspect of the symphysis. With manual retraction of the bladder to one side, the first laparotomy pad is placed around the bladder and into the depth of the pelvic space. A ringed forceps or Cobb elevator is used to push this first pack down to the sacroiliac joint. Successive packs (#2 and #3) are placed around the bladder, in the upside down U shape of the pelvic space comprising the paravesicle and retropubic space. The sequence is then repeated on the opposite side until both sides of the pelvis are packed. This typically requires six laparotomy pads, but up to nine pads may be necessary for effective hemorrhage control. In the pediatric patients, two packs on each side of the pelvis may be all that is necessary to accomplish hemostasis. The midline fascia is then closed with a running large monofilament suture followed by skin closure with staples.

There are some key technical points that facilitate effective and expeditious PPP. First, collaboration with the orthopedic team is critical. Typically external fixation occurs prior to PPP. If so, optimal location of the external fixation frame should be discussed. The anterior bar or the external fixator should be positioned so that there is access for the PPP incision. Typically this results in a cephalad orientation of the bar. Alternatively, if a laparotomy is required, the bar should be positioned low over the upper thighs for access to both the abdomen and pelvic spaces. The second key consideration is the need for laparotomy. Many of these patients require intervention for intra-abdominal hemorrhage based upon FAST imaging. The laparotomy and PPP incisions should be kept separate (Fig. 15.4); combining the incisions into a single long midline opens the pelvic space into the peritoneal space and makes PPP much less effective. Finally, patients may have associated urethral injuries. At the time of PPP, suprapubic catheters can rapidly be placed for bladder decompression and are typically placed via a separate stab incision lateral to the PPP incision (Fig. 15.5). Following pelvic stabilization and PPP, the abdomen is reassessed using physiologic parameters and ultrasound to ensure laparotomy is not necessary for bleeding or the abdominal compartment syndrome.

Angioembolization is used as an adjunct for pelvic fracture-related hemorrhage control following PPP. With only 13% of PPP patients requiring angioembolization for arterial bleeding following PPP [17], transfusion requirements post-packing dictate which patients need this invasive, resource-intensive intervention. Current algorithms suggest that once the patient's coagulopathy is corrected, if more than four units of red cells are transfused in the first 12 h postoperatively, these patients should

Fig. 15.4 The laparotomy and PPP incisions are separate; the PPP incision is seen stapled just beneath the external fixator with a widely open midline laparotomy incision

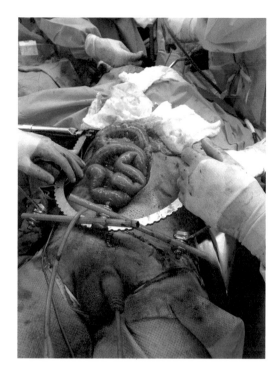

Fig. 15.5 Suprapubic catheters are placed via a separate stab incision lateral to the PPP incision

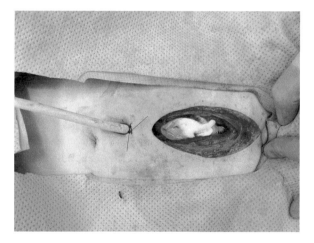

undergo diagnostic angiography (Fig. 15.1). Only those patients with a documented blush should undergo selective embolization with Gelfoam. Empiric embolization of bilateral internal iliac arteries is rarely indicated.

Following physiologic restoration in the ICU, the patient is returned to the operating room for pelvic pack removal between 24 and 48 h postinjury. Coagulopathy must be corrected prior to operative return to prevent need for repacking of the pelvis. Repacking of the pelvis is associated with an increase in infectious complications from 6% to 47% [17] and hence should be avoided. Individual ligation of small vessels, coagulation of bleeders, and use of topical anticoagulants are used to address minor hemorrhage upon pack removal. Following pack removal and hemostasis, the pelvic space is irrigated and closed. Definitive orthopedic fixation of the symphysis, if necessary, is often delayed to a separate procedure.

Take-Home Points
1. The vast majority of patients delivered to the emergency department (ED) with a pelvic fracture are hemodynamically stable; 5–10% of patients arrive in hemorrhagic shock and represent a unique challenge for the trauma team.
2. Many patients with pelvic fractures will sustain concomitant life-threatening injuries: 20% have thoracic trauma, 17% have head injury, 8% have significant liver or spleen trauma, and 8% have >2 long bone fracture.
3. Injuries that necessitate early recognition in patients with pelvic fractures include bladder, urethral, rectal, vaginal, external iliac arterial, and lumbosacral nerve injuries.
4. The focus in patients with unstable pelvic fractures is rapid hemorrhage control; this can be accomplished with resuscitative endovascular aortic balloon occlusion of the aorta (REBOA) and peritoneal pelvic packing in combination with the accepted standards of ED pelvic binding and goal-directed hemostasis with early blood components.
5. Immediate percutaneous common femoral arterial cannulation with a 7 French Pinnacle Precision Access System (Terumo Medical, Elkton, MD) is performed on patients in shock (SBP < 90 mmHg) with ultrasound guidance. Partial responders with systolic blood pressure less than 80 mmHg are treated by placement of the REBOA catheter through the femoral artery sheath.
6. Because 85% of pelvic fracture related bleeding is venous or bony in origin, hemorrhage can be tamponaded within the retroperitoneal space with preperitoneal pelvic packing.
7. The indication for peritoneal pelvic packing/external fixation is hypotension despite two units of red cell transfusion.
8. Angioembolization is used as an adjunct for pelvic fracture-related hemorrhage control following PPP with 13% requiring this intervention; once the patient's coagulopathy is corrected, if more than four units of red cells are transfused in the first 12 hours postoperatively, patients should undergo diagnostic angiography.

Don't play poker with someone else's chips. Harlan Stone

References

1. Costantini TW, Coimbra R, Holcomb JB, AAST Pelvic Fracture Study Group, et al. Current management of hemorrhage from severe pelvic fractures: results of an American Association for the Surgery of Trauma multi-institutional trial. J Trauma Acute Care Surg. 2016;80(5):717–25.

2. Cullinane DC, Schiller HJ, Zielinski MD, et al. Eastern Association for the Surgery of trauma practice management guidelines for hemorrhage in pelvic fracture--update and systematic review. J Trauma. 2011;71(6):1850–68.
3. Gonzalez E, Moore EE, Moore HB, et al. Goal-directed hemostatic resuscitation of trauma-induced coagulopathy: a pragmatic randomized clinical trial comparing a viscoelastic assay to conventional coagulation assays. Ann Surg. 2016;263(6):1051–9.
4. Giannoudis PV, Grotz MR, Tzioupis C, et al. Prevalence of pelvic fractures, associated injuries, and mortality: the United Kingdom perspective. J Trauma. 2007;63:875.
5. Biffl WL, Fox CJ, Moore EE. The role of REBOA in the control of exsanguinating torso hemorrhage. J Trauma Acute Care Surg. 2015;78(5):1054–8.
6. Rasmussen TE, DuBose JJ, Asensio JA, et al. Tourniquets, vascular shunts, and endovascular technologies: esoteric or essential? A report from the 2011 AAST military liaison panel. J Trauma Acute Care Surg. 2012;73(1):282–5.
7. Stannard A, Eliason JL, Rasmussen TE. Resuscitative endovascular balloon occlusion of the aorta (REBOA) as an adjunct for hemorrhagic shock. J Trauma Acute Care Surg. 2011;71(6):1869–72.
8. Azizzadeh A, Ray HM, Dubose JJ, et al. Outcomes of endovascular repair for patients with blunt traumatic aortic injury. J Trauma Acute Care Surg. 2014;76(2):510–6.
9. du Toit DF, Lambrechts AV, Stark H, Warren BL. Long-term results of stent graft treatment of subclavian artery injuries: management of choice for stable patients? J Vasc Surg. 2008;47(4):739–43.
10. Reuben BC, Whitten MG, Sarfati M, Kraiss LW. Increasing use of endovascular therapy in acute arterial injuries: analysis of the National Trauma Data Bank. J Vasc Surg. 2007;46(6):1222–6.
11. Holcomb JB. Methods for improved hemorrhage control. Crit Care. 2004;8(Suppl 2):S57.
12. Martinelli T, Thony F, Declety P, et al. Intra-aortic balloon occlusion to salvage patients with life-threatening hemorrhagic shocks from pelvic fractures. J Trauma. 2010;68:942–8.
13. Stahel PF, Mauffrey C, Smith WR, et al. External fixation for acute pelvic ring injuries: decision making and technical options. J Trauma Acute Care Surg. 2013;75:882–7.
14. Pohlmann T, Gansslen A, Bosch U, Tscherne H. The technique of packing for control of hemorrhage in complex pelvis fractures. Tech Orthop. 1995;9:267–70.
15. Ertel W, Keel M, Eid K, et al. Control of severe hemorrhage using c-clamp and pelvic packing in multiply injured patients with pelvic ring disruption. J Orthop Trauma. 2001;15(7):468–74.
16. Cothren CC, Osborn PM, Moore EE, et al. Preperitoneal pelvic packing for hemodynamically unstable pelvic fractures: a paradigm shift. J Trauma. 2007;62:834–42.
17. Burlew CC, Moore EE, Smith WR, et al. Preperitoneal pelvic packing/external fixation with secondary angioembolization: optimal care for life-threatening hemorrhage from unstable pelvic fractures. J Am Coll Surg. 2011;212:628–37.

Chapter 16
Vascular Damage Control Techniques: What Do I Do When All Else Fails?

Chad G. Ball

Case Scenario

A 27-year-old female sustains a single large-caliber gunshot wound and presents in extremis. Upon emergent exploration, she has a number of injuries, but it quickly becomes clear that the missile has transected her superior mesenteric artery cleanly off of her aorta. The bleeding is tremendous, and the vascular surgeon is located 100 miles away…

Damage control is a Navy term defined as "the capacity of a ship to absorb damage and maintain mission integrity" [1]. Although the adaption of this term to the field of traumatology can be credited to Dr. Schwab and colleagues in 1993 [2], its dominant principles are more accurately rooted in Dr. Lucas and Ledgerwood's 1976 address to the American Association for the Surgery of Trauma [3]. More specifically, they described a small series of patients who underwent sponge-based packing of major liver injuries [3]. This concept was reiterated shortly thereafter by Calne [4], as well as Feliciano and Mattox [5] in 1979 and 1981, respectively. Despite these small series outlining the success of perihepatic packing, the visionary extrapolation of this principle to patients with multiple concurrent life-threatening injuries and major coagulopathy was not published until 1983 [6]. Harlan Stone retrospectively described 31 patients who developed major bleeding diatheses [6].

The natural extension and further development of DCS have been damage control *resuscitation* (DCR) [7–11]. This concept includes not only DCS but also the early initiation of blood product transfusions and massive transfusion protocols, reduced crystalloid fluid administration, permissive hypotension in selected populations, and immediate hemorrhage control (whether operative or angiographic). In other words, DCR is a structured intervention that is mobile and can be delivered to

C.G. Ball, MD, MSc, FRCSC, FACS (✉)
Hepatobiliary and Pancreatic Surgery, Trauma and Acute Care Surgery, University of Calgary, Foothills Medical Centre, Calgary, AB, Canada
e-mail: ball.chad@gmail.com

© Springer International Publishing AG 2018   193
C.G. Ball, E. Dixon (eds.), *Treatment of Ongoing Hemorrhage*,
DOI 10.1007/978-3-319-63495-1_16

Table 16.1 Massive transfusion protocol: package contents

Package	PRBCs	Plasma	Platelets	Cryoprecipitate
Initiation	6 units (UD/TS)	6 units (UD)		
1 (0.5 h)	6 units (UD/TS)	6 units (UD)	1 apheresis[a]	
2 (1 h)	6 units (UD/TS)	6 units (TS)		20 units
3 (1. 5 h)[b]	6 units (UD/TS)	6 units (TS)	1 apheresis[a]	
4 (2 h)	6 units (UD/TS)	6 units (TS)		10 units
5 (2.5 h)	6 units (UD/TS)	6 units (TS)	1 apheresis[a]	
6 (3 h)[c]	6 units (UD/TS)	6 units (TS)		10 units

PRBCs packed red blood cells, *UD* universal donor, *TS* type specific
PRBCs and plasma can be doubled to 12 units each per cycle by request
[a]One apheresis unit of platelets considered to equal 8–10 standard units
[b]Recombinant factor VIIa may be used at attending physician discretion (Dose, 3.6 mg; one repeat dose as needed in 30 min)
[c]If protocol is still active, alternate packages identical to packages 5 and 6 until protocol is terminated

Table 16.2 Open abdomen coverage techniques

Skin only	Polypropylene mesh
Towel clip	Polyglycolic/polyglactic acid mesh
Silastic sheet	Polytetrafluoroethylene mesh
Bogota bag	Parachute silk
3-liter genitourinary bag	Hydrogel/Aquacel
Steri-drape/x-ray cassette	Ioban
Zippers	Vacuum pack
Slide fasteners	Abdominal wound VAC
Velcro analogue/Wittmann	Bioprosthetics

a critically ill patient in any location (emergency department, interventional radiology suite, operating theater, and/or intensive care unit). Regardless of their destination, arresting hemorrhage, restoring blood volume, and correcting coagulopathy are ongoing. Preceding chapters within this textbook have outlined the mechanics of massive transfusion and permissive hypotension. Both remain critical to the successful completion of damage control vascular surgery in the patient with ongoing massive hemorrhage (Tables 16.1 and 16.2).

Vascular Damage Control Surgery (DCS) Indications

The maturation of DCS has led to fundamental tenants that include (1) arresting surgical hemorrhage, (2) containment of gastrointestinal spillage, (3) surgical sponge insertion, and (4) temporary abdominal closure. This sequence is followed by immediate transfer to the intensive care unit with subsequent rewarming, correction of coagulopathy, and hemodynamic stabilization. Return to the operating theater is then pursued 6–48 h later for a planned re-exploration that includes definitive repair and primary fascial closure if possible. It is clear that the DCS approach leads to improved survival for both blunt and penetrating injures in patients who are approaching physiologic exhaustion [12].

Despite the clear utility of DCS, its widespread propagation throughout the trauma community has led to a clear overutilization of this technique. More specifically, multiple injured patients who are *not* approaching physiologic exhaustion are often exposed to the potential risks associated with open abdomens. As a result, the pertinent question remains: who needs DCS? The succinct response is "patients who are more likely to die from uncorrected shock states than from failure to complete organ repairs." In essence, these are metabolic cripples who continue to suffer the sequelae of tissue shock that is manifested as *persistent* hypothermia, *persistent* metabolic acidosis, and nonmechanical (i.e., nonsurgical) bleeding. More specifically, DCS triggers include core temperature <35 °C, pH < 7.2, base deficit > −15, and/or significant coagulopathies [13–16]. It must be emphasized however that not even all patients with initial physiologic deficits as significant as these values mandate DCS[17–33]. With rapid arrest of hemorrhage, as well as ongoing resuscitation, some patients will improve dramatically in all parameters on repeated intraoperative blood gases. These patients stabilize and begin to recover. It should also be stated that patients with multiple intra-abdominal injuries are not always in metabolic failure.

Vascular Damage Control Techniques

Although it is clear that arresting ongoing hemorrhage is the most crucial of damage control tenants, *vascular* damage control has been traditionally limited to vessel ligation. More recently, however, balloon catheter tamponade and temporary intravascular shunts (TIVS) have increased in popularity. The impressive utility of balloon catheters for tamponade of exsanguinating hemorrhage has a long history dating back more than 50 years [34]. Although this technique was originally described for esophageal varices [35], it was quickly extended to patients with traumatic vascular and solid organ injuries [36]. Since the initial treatment of an iliac arteriovenous lesion in 1960 [3], balloon catheters have also been used for cardiac [37], aortic [38], pelvic vascular [39], neck (carotid, vertebral, and jugular vessels) [40, 41], abdominal vascular [42], hepatic vascular [43], subclavian [44], vertebral [34], and facial vascular trauma [45]. While this technique was originally intended as an intraoperative endovascular tool [34], it has since been employed as an emergency room maneuver with the balloon being placed outside of the lumen of the injured vessel [46, 47].

Fig. 16.1 Blakemore
occlusion balloon

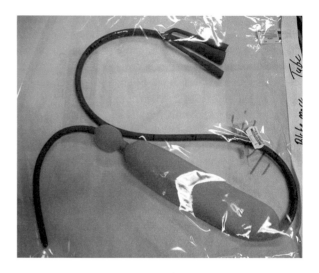

Fig. 16.2 Red rubber/
Penrose occlusion balloon

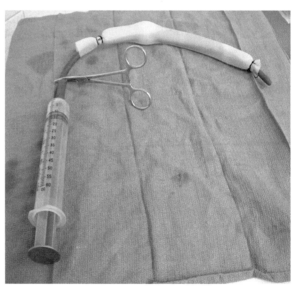

Balloon Catheter Tamponade

Modern indications for this damage control technique are limited. This is primarily because routine methods for controlling hemorrhage, such as direct pressure, are typically successful. As a result, indications for catheter tamponade include (1) inaccessible (or difficult to access) major vascular injuries, (2) large cardiac injuries, and (3) deep solid organ parenchymal hemorrhage (liver and lung) [34, 37]. The specific type of balloon catheter (Foley, Fogarty, Blakemore, or Penrose with Red Rubber Robinson) (Figs. 16.1 and 16.2), as well as the duration of indwelling,

Fig. 16.3 Cervical Foley catheter balloon occlusion

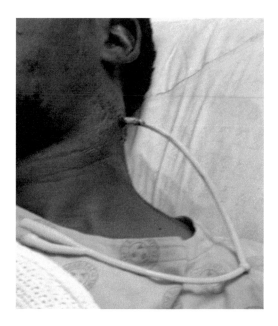

can vary significantly. The take-home message is to ensure a selection of various catheters is available in a central kit that is easily accessible within the operating theater and emergency department. In its purest essence, balloon catheter tamponade is a valuable tool for damage control of exsanguinating hemorrhage when direct pressure fails or tourniquets are not applicable. It can be employed in multiple anatomic regions and for variable patterns of injury.

The technical nuances and skill required to successfully insert a balloon catheter into a wound or organ with ongoing hemorrhage are relatively minimal. Think of the balloon and the wound as a geometric puzzle. Select the type of balloon that you think will best fit within the space. This may range from a Foley (penetrating neck wound) to a Blakemore (central hepatic gunshot wound) to a Fogarty (insertion into the internal carotid artery when it is sheared off of the mastoid via a penetrating wound) catheter (Figs. 16.3, 16.4, 16.5, 16.6, and 16.7). The important point is to make the decision to insert the balloon early after an initial one or maximum of two other techniques have failed. An experienced clinician will usually recognize wound dynamics and geometry and select the appropriate balloon as a primary hemostatic choice. Once the catheter is inserted into the wound, it should be gently inflated with water. If the hemorrhage stops, then the catheter should be either tied off with a knot or clamped to prevent both movement and blood flow through some balloon devices (i.e., Foley). If the catheter is left in place for any significant length of time, it should be secured with copious amounts of tape and warning labels begging all caregivers not to touch the catheter itself. If the ongoing hemorrhage is not stopped by the initial insertion of the catheter, there is one of two potential problems: (1) you've used the wrong balloon for the geometry of the wound, or (2) the balloon needs to be repositioned. In the second scenario, desufflate the balloon and either

Fig. 16.4 Cervical Foley
catheter balloon occlusion

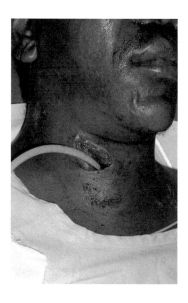

Fig. 16.5 Balloon
occlusion for central
hepatic gunshot wound

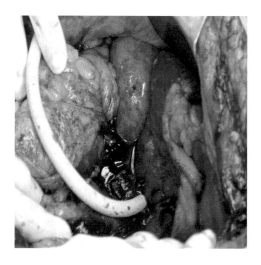

advance or retract it and then reinflate it again. This nuanced cycle may be required
more than once. Don't be discouraged!! If the skin wound is too large to keep the
catheter contained and it continues to pop out of the wound (e.g., neck), then close
the skin around the tube itself (i.e., similar to a chest tube suture) to lock it into
place. As previously mentioned, a successfully placed balloon catheter can remain
in place for an extended duration (i.e., prolonged interval for central hepatic gunshot
wounds).

Fig. 16.6 Deflation of balloon occlusion for central hepatic gunshot wound

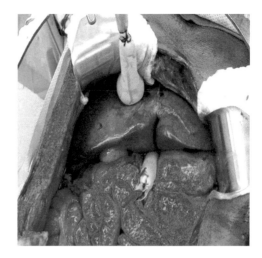

Fig. 16.7 Foley catheter balloon occlusion of the severed internal carotid artery at the skull base

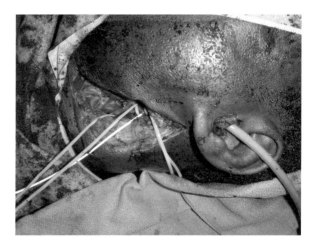

Temporary Intravascular Shunts

Temporary intravascular shunts (TIVS) are intraluminal synthetic conduits that offer nonpermanent maintenance of arterial inflow and/or venous outflow [48] (Figs. 16.8 and 16.9). As a result, they are frequently life- and limb-saving when patient physiology is hostile. By bridging a damaged vessel and maintaining blood flow, they address both acute hemorrhage and critical warm ischemia of distal organs and limbs. Although Eger and colleagues are commonly credited for pioneering the use of TIVS in modern vascular trauma [49], this technique was initially employed by Carrel in animal experiments [50]. The first documented use in humans occurred in 1915 when Tuffier employed paraffin-coated silver tubes to bridge

Fig. 16.8 Vascular shunt
of the iliac artery and vein

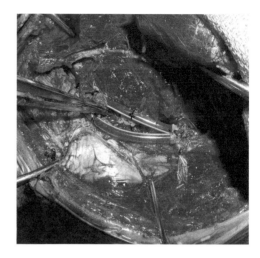

Fig. 16.9 Vascular shunt
of the iliac artery and
ureterostomy intubation

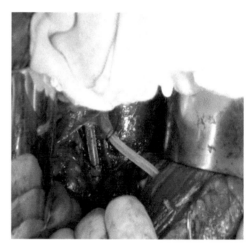

injured arteries [51]. This technique evolved from glass to plastic conduits in World
War II [52] and continues to vary both in structure and material among today's
surgeons [53].

Modern indications for TIVS include (1) replantation, (2) open extremity fractures with concurrent extensive soft tissue loss and arterial injury (Gustilo IIIC)
(Fig. 16.10), (3) peripheral vascular damage control, (4) truncal vascular damage
control (Fig. 16.11), and (5) temporary stabilization prior to transport [48, 54].
While the understanding of TIVS use for military and civilian settings is increasing
[53], the optimal shunt material, dwell time, and anticoagulation requirements
remain poorly studied. It can be noted however that TIVS are remarkably durable
and rarely clot off unless they (1) are too small (diameter), (2) kink because of
inappropriate length, and/or (3) are placed in an extremity without appropriate (or
shunted) venous outflow (venous hypertension leads to arterial thrombosis) [54].

Fig. 16.10 Vascular shunt in a Gustilo IIIC injury

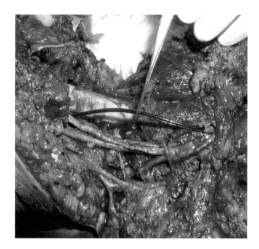

Fig. 16.11 Vascular shunt of the superior mesenteric artery

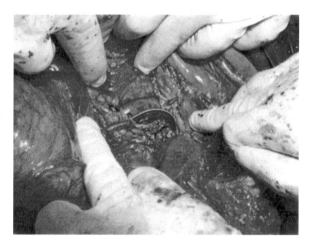

Despite often talking about TIVS in the context of penetrating mechanisms, this technique is also excellent for numerous blunt trauma scenarios [55]. More specifically, they are excellent as a temporizing vascular maneuver to provide distal flow to a limb while orthopedic injuries are assessed and fixated (which are then subsequently followed by an appropriate vascular reconstruction if the patient's physiology allows). The use of TIVS for this scenario is well recognized and documented to significantly reduce the rate of amputation. In addition to using TIVS in blunt-injured patients, the NTDB also indicates this technique is being performed relatively uncommonly across a wide range of hospitals [55]. This underutilization is surprising given their simplicity.

Similar to balloon catheters, various sizes and types of tubes can be used as a TIVS. This ranges from argyle carotid shunts to chest tubes (Figs. 16.12 and 16.13). As a result, an array of tube options should be kept together in a kit that is easily accessible in the operating theater. The important principles when selecting a tube for insertion as a TIVS are to ensure (1) it is not undersized with regard to diameter,

Fig. 16.12 Javid vascular shunts

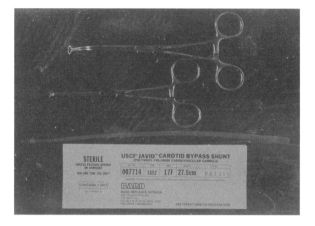

Fig. 16.13 Pruitt vascular shunts

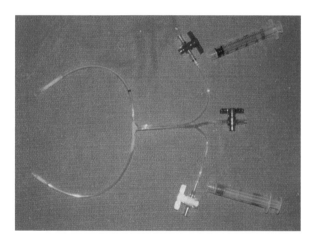

(2) it will not become kinked given its positioning (even in prolonged transport), and (3) it is stiff enough to avoid issue #2. Once inserted into the vessel in an in-line manner, the TIVS can be locked into place via either silk ties or double-vessel loops that are tightened/locked with clips. If silk ties are selected, it must be remembered that the vessel itself will need to be trimmed back proximal to the silk to ensure there is no ischemia at the time of the reconstruction. This may become a problem for the surgeon in areas where every bit of vessel length is critical. The authors utilize shorter shunt lengths in scenarios where the patient is expected to remain within the same institution but will switch to using a longer TIVS with an intentional loop in cases where prehospital transport is subsequently required. This allows improved fixation to the patient, as well as the ability to confirm flow/patency through the tube during transport scenarios. It should also be reemphasized that TIVS do not require systemic anticoagulation to remain patent. If the tube is sized correctly, it can remain indwelling without concern for a prolonged period of time (i.e., without systemic anticoagulation or heparin-bonded tubing). In summary, these tubes are often both life- and limb-saving!

Take-Home Points
1. Be sure your patient actually needs a damage control procedure!
2. Vascular shunts (TIVS) are simple and save lives and limbs.
3. Balloons are even simpler and save lives all day every day!!
4. Create a ready-to-go box in your operating theater with a multitude of shunts and balloons.
5. Both shunts and balloons are underutilized, so don't forget about them!!

There are cemeteries full of people who are dead because they were not explored quickly enough for penetrating trauma. Harlan Stone

References

1. Manual for Naval warfare. United States of America Navy. 1996.
2. Rotondo MF, Schwab CW, McGonigal MD, Phillips GR 3rd, Fruchterman TM, Kauder DR, et al. Damage control: an approach for improved survival in exsanguinating penetrating abdominal injury. J Trauma. 1993;35:375–83.
3. Lucas CE, Ledgerwood AM. Prospective evaluation of hemostatic techniques for liver injuries. J Trauma. 1976;16:442–51.
4. Calne RY, McMaster P, Pentlow BD. The treatment of major liver trauma by primary packing with transfer of the patient for definitive treatment. Br J Surg. 1979;66:338–9.
5. Feliciano DV, Mattox KL, Jordan GL Jr. Intra-abdominal packing for control of hepatic hemorrhage: a reappraisal. J Trauma. 1981;21:285–90.
6. Stone HH, Strom PR, Mullins RJ. Management of the major coagulopathy with onset during laparotomy. Ann Surg. 1983;197:532–5.
7. Firoozmand E, Velmahos GC. Extending damage control principles to the neck. J Trauma. 2000;48:541.
8. Granchi T, Schmittling Z, Vasquez J, Schreiber M, Wall M. Prolonged use of intraluminal arterial shunts without systemic anticoagulation. Am J Surg. 2000;180:493–6.
9. Scalea TM, Boswell SA, Scott JD, Mitchell KA, Kramer ME, Pollak AN, et al. External fixation as a bridge to nailing for patients with multiple injuries and with femur fractures: damage control orthopedics. J Trauma. 2000;48:613–23.
10. Vargo DJ, Battistella FD. Abbreviated thoracotomy and temporary chest closure: an application of damage control after thoracic trauma. Arch Surg. 2001;136:21–4.
11. Holcomb JB, Helling TS, Hirshber A. Military, civilian and rural application of the damage control philosophy. Mil Med. 2001;166:490–3.
12. Nicholas JM, Rix EP, Easley KA, Feliciano DV, Cava RA, Ingram WL, et al. Changing patterns in the management of penetrating abdominal trauma: the more things change, the more they stay the same. J Trauma. 2003;55:1095–108.
13. Lier H, Krep H, Schroeder S, Stuber F. The influence of acidosis, hypocalcemia, anemia, and hypothermia on functional hemostasis in trauma. J Trauma. 2008;65:951–60.
14. Wyrzykowski AD, Feliciano DV. Trauma damage control. In: Feliciano DV, Mattox KL, Moore EE, editors. Trauma. 6th ed. New York: McGraw-Hill Medical; 2008. p. 851–70.
15. Cushman JG, Feliciano DV, Renz BM, Ingram WL, Ansley JD, Clark WS, et al. Iliac vessel injury: operative physiology related to outcome. J Trauma. 1997;42:1033–40.
16. Holcomb JB, Jenkins D, Rhee P, Johannigman J, Mahoney P, Mehta S, et al. Damage control resuscitation: directly addressing the early coagulopathy of trauma. J Trauma. 2007;62:307–10.
17. Bickell WH, Wall MJ Jr, Pepe PE, Martin RR, Ginger VF, Allen MK, et al. Immediate versus delayed fluid resuscitation for hypotensive patients with penetrating torso injuries. N Engl J Med. 1994;27:1105–9.

18. Morrison CA, Carrick MM, Norman MA, et al. Hypotensive resuscitation strategy reduces transfusion requirements and severe postoperative coagulopathy in trauma patients with hemorrhagic shock: preliminary results of a randomized controlled trial. J Trauma. 2011;70:652–63.
19. Como JJ, Dutton RP, Scalea TM, Edelman BB, Hess JR. Blood transfusion rates in the care of acute trauma. Transfusion. 2004;44:809–13.
20. Brohi K, Singh J, Hern M, Coats T. Acute traumatic coagulopathy. J Trauma. 2003;54:1127–30.
21. Hess JR, Brohi K, Dutton RP, Hauser CJ, Holcomb JB, Kluger Y, et al. The coagulopathy of trauma: a review of mechanisms. J Trauma. 2008;65:748–54.
22. Borgman MA, Spinella PC, Perkins JG, Grathwohl KW, Repine T, Beekley AC, et al. The ratio of blood products transfuse affects mortality in patients receiving massive transfusions at a combat support hospital. J Trauma. 2007;64:805–13.
23. Dente CJ, Shaz BH, Nicholas JM, Harris RS, Wyrzykowski AD, Patel S, et al. Improvements in early mortality and coagulopathy are sustained better in patients with blunt trauma after institution of a massive transfusion protocol in a civilian level I trauma center. J Trauma. 2009;66:1616–24.
24. Sheldon GF, Lim RC, Blaisdell FW. The use of fresh blood in the treatment of critically injured patients. J Trauma. 1975;15:670–7.
25. O'Keeffe T, Refaai M, Tchorz K, Forestner JE, Sarode R. A massive transfusion protocol to decrease blood component use and cost. Arch Surg. 2008;143:686–90.
26. Snyder CW, Weinberg JA, McGwin G Jr, Melton SM, George RL, Reiff DA, et al. The relationship of blood product ratio to mortality: survival benefit or survival bias? J Trauma. 2009;66:358–62.
27. Park PK, Cannon JW, Ye W, Blackbourne LH, Holcomb JB, Beninati W, et al. Transfusion strategies and development of acute respiratory distress syndrome in combat casualty care. J Trauma Acute Care Surg. 2013;75(S):S238–46.
28. Inaba K, Branco BC, Rhee P, et al. Impact of plasma transfusion in trauma patients who do not require massive transfusion. J Am Coll Surg. 2010;210:957–65.
29. Sharpe JP, Weinberg JA, Magnotti LJ, Fabian TC, Croce MA. Does plasma transfusion portend pulmonary dysfunction? A tale of two ratios. J Trauma Acute Care Surg. 2013;75:32–6.
30. Cotton BA, Guy JS, Morris JA, Abumrad NN. Cellular, metabolic, and systemic consequences of aggressive fluid resuscitation strategies. Shock. 2006;26:115–21.
31. Rhee P, Koustova E, Alam HB. Searching for the optimal resuscitation method: recommendations for the initial fluid resuscitation of combat casualties. J Trauma. 2003;54:S52.
32. Pruitt BA Jr. Protection for excessive resuscitation: "pushing the pendulum back". J Trauma. 2000;49:567–8.
33. Ball CG, Kirkpatrick AW. Intra-abdominal hypertension and the abdominal compartment syndrome. Scand J Surg. 2007;96:197–204.
34. Feliciano DV, Burch JM, Mattox KL, Bitondo CG, Fields G. Balloon catheter tamponade in cardiovascular wounds. Am J Surg. 1990;160:583–7.
35. Myhre JR. Balloon tamponade of hemorrhagic esophageal varices. Tidsskr Nor Laegeforen. 1958;78:511–3.
36. Taylor H, Williams E. Arteriovenous fistula following disk surgery. Br J Surg. 1962;50:47–50.
37. Pearce CW, McCool E, Schmidt FE. Control of bleeding from cardiovascular wounds: balloon catheter tamponade. Ann Surg. 1966;166:257–9.
38. Foster JH, Morgan CV, Threlkel JB. Proximal control of aorta with a balloon catheter. Surg Gynecol Obstet. 1971;132:693–4.
39. Sheldon GF, Winestock DP. Hemorrhage from open pelvic fracture controlled intraoperatively with balloon catheter. J Trauma. 1978;18:68–70.
40. Belkin M, Dunton R, Crombie HD, Lowe R. Preoperative percutaneous intraluminal balloon catheter control of major arterial hemorrhage. J Trauma. 1988;28:548–50.
41. Brendahan J, Swanepoel E, Muller R. Tamponade of vertebral artery bleeding by Foley's catheter balloon. Injury. 1994;25:473–4.

42. Smiley K, Perry MO. Balloon catheter tamponade of major vascular wounds. Am J Surg. 1971;121:326–7.
43. Morimoto RY, Birolini D, Junqueira AR Jr, Poggetti R, Horita LT. Balloon tamponade for transfixing lesions of the liver. Surg Gynecol Obstet. 1987;164:87–8.
44. DiGiacomo JC, Rotondo MF, Schwab CW. Transcutaneous balloon catheter tamponade for definitive control of subclavian venous injuries: case reports. J Trauma. 1994;37:111–3.
45. Sing RF, Sue SR, Reilly PM. Balloon catheter tamponade of exsanguinating facial hemorrhage: a case report. J Emerg Med. 1998;16:601–2.
46. Navsaria P, Thoma M, Nicol A. Foley catheter balloon tamponade for life-threatening hemorrhage in penetrating neck trauma. World J Surg. 2006;30:1265–8.
47. Ball CG, Wyrzykowski AD, Nicholas JM, Rozycki GS, Feliciano DV. A decade's experience with balloon catheter tamponade for the emergency control of hemorrhage. J Trauma. 2011;70:330–3.
48. Frykberg ER, Schinco MA. Peripheral vascular injury. In: Feliciano DV, Mattox KL, Moore EE, editors. Trauma. 6th ed. New York: McGraw-Hill Medical; 2008. p. 956–7.
49. Eger M, Golcman L, Goldstein A, Hirsch M. The use of a temporary shunt in the management of arterial vascular injuries. Surg Gynecol Obstet. 1971;132:67–70.
50. Makins GH. Gunshot injuries to the blood vessels. London: Simpkin, Marshall, Hamilton, Kent & Co; 1919. p. 109–11.
51. Tuffier JT. French surgery in 1915. Br J Surg. 1916;4:420–32.
52. Matheson NM, Murray G. Recent advances and experimental work in conservative vascular surgery. In: Bailey H, editor. Surgery of modern warfare, vol. 1. Baltimore: Williams and Wilkins; 1941. p. 324–7.
53. Ding W, Wu X, Li J. Temporary intravascular shunts used as a damage control surgery adjunct in complex vascular injury: collective review. Injury. 2008;39:970–7.
54. Ball CG, Feliciano DV. Damage control techniques for common and external iliac artery injuries: have temporary intravascular shunts replaced the need for ligation? J Trauma. 2010;68:1117–20.
55. Ball CG, Kirkpatrick AW, Rajani RR, Wyrzykowski AD, Dente CJ, Vercruysse GA, et al. Temporary intravascular shunts (TIVS): when are we really using them according to the NTDB? Am Surg. 2009;75:605–7.

Chapter 17
Extremity Trauma Hemorrhage: More than Just a Tourniquet

Nathan R. Manley and Martin A. Croce

Case Scenario

A 55-year-old farmer arrives with an extremely complex laceration of his left leg up to his hip after falling into a bailer. You quickly identify the Gustilo 3C nature of the wound and immediately transfer him to the operating theater in the company of your orthopedic and plastic surgical colleagues…

Initial Management

The initial management of hemorrhage in the extremity begins with direct pressure over obvious bleeding and elevation of the extremity. A pressure dressing using a variety of materials can be applied during transport to the trauma center or in route to the operating room. If direct pressure fails, a tourniquet can be applied proximal to the bleeding, especially in the context of exsanguinating hemorrhage in the unstable patient. The overall condition of the patient, including concomitant injuries to the head, chest, and abdomen, will dictate the priority of exploration and repair. A primary survey should be completed, and the patient should be actively resuscitated with fluid and blood as necessary to maintain systemic perfusion (life over limb).

N.R. Manley, MD, MPH (✉) • M.A. Croce, MD
Department of Surgery, University of Tennessee Health Science Center, Memphis, TN, USA
e-mail: nmanley1@uthsc.edu

© Springer International Publishing AG 2018
C.G. Ball, E. Dixon (eds.), *Treatment of Ongoing Hemorrhage*,
DOI 10.1007/978-3-319-63495-1_17

Table 17.1 Vascular injuries associated with fractures and dislocations

Orthopedic injury	Vascular injury
Anterior shoulder dislocation	Axillary artery
Supracondylar humeral fracture	Brachial artery
Supracondylar femur fracture	Popliteal artery
Posterior knee dislocation	
Tibial plateau fracture	Popliteal artery, tibioperoneal trunk

Table 17.2 Hard signs of arterial injury

Active hemorrhage
Absent distal pulses
Expanding, pulsatile hematoma
Palpable thrill or audible bruit
Five Ps: pain, pallor, paralysis, paresthesias, poikilothermia

Physical Exam

It is important to perform and document baseline vascular and neurologic examinations to serve as a point of comparison after surgical exploration and repair. In these patients, an abnormal neurologic examination is not necessarily indicative of concomitant nerve injury. The neurologic dysfunction may be a manifestation of ischemia from the vascular injury, so prompt control and revascularization are paramount to preserve function. Certain orthopedic injuries should raise suspicion for specific vascular injuries (Table 17.1).

Vascular Examination

Pulses should be checked in all four extremities, paying special attention to any discrepancies between the injured and uninjured limb. A Doppler should be available and utilized if pulses are not palpable. If there is a penetrating wound to the lower extremity, perform ankle-brachial indices (ABIs) if time and the patient's condition allow. In addition to active hemorrhage, other hard signs of arterial injury indicate immediate operative exploration for more subtle trauma and are summarized in Table 17.2. With injuries to the forearm, it is important to perform an Allen's test to confirm patent flow in the collateral artery, especially if considering ligation.

Neurologic Examination

A motor and sensory exam should be performed in the injured extremity and compared to the uninjured side if the patient is awake and alert. Remember that vascular injuries can cause peripheral nerve ischemia and that nerve injury can only be excluded if deficits persist after vascular repair or if the nerve is intact at exploration.

General Principles of Exploration, Exposure, and Repair

Once obvious bleeding has been controlled and a baseline vascular and neurologic exam documented, the next step is isolating the source and deciding if the vein, artery, or both have been injured. This can be completed in the trauma bay, but when faced with hard signs of vascular injury, do not delay transfer to the OR. The color of the blood (bright red vs dark red) and the nature of the bleeding (pulsatile vs nonpulsatile) can offer important clues to differentiate arterial and venous injury but can be misleading in a patient who is under-resuscitated or in extremis. Direct visualization of the injury and knowledge of limb-specific anatomy are crucial. Direct pressure should be maintained during sterile preparation and until the injured vessel can be identified and isolated.

Basic Operative Principles for Arterial Injuries

Always prep and drape an uninjured lower extremity in anticipation of harvesting a saphenous vein to serve as an interposition graft. Vascular repair and reperfusion of the extremity should take precedence over any other repair once threats to life in the primary survey are under control. Once exposed, obtain proximal and distal control of the injured vessel. An intraluminal catheter balloon can be used as an adjunct to obtain proximal control. Thoroughly examine the injured vessel. Systemic heparinization should be given by anesthesia prior to repair. Heparin can be weight based or can be given in doses of 2500–5000 units per hour. Ideally, if resources permit, the activated clotting time (ACT) should be followed routinely and dictate additional doses of heparin.

Primary or lateral repair of arteries should be done if possible; typically, this is an option only with stab wounds. Pay special attention to any narrowing of the lumen after repair.

If the artery is partially or completely transected, debride back to the healthy tissue on proximal and distal ends, and perform a primary anastomosis if there is not undue tension. Remember to perform balloon catheter thrombectomy both proximally and distally prior to anastomosis. It is also important to mobilize both

Table 17.3 Arteries and veins that can be ligated

Injury	Best mode of action	
Brachial artery	1. Repair	2. Can ligate if distal to profunda brachii – The elbow has rich collateral blood supply
Radial and ulnar arteries	1. Repair	2. Can ligate but need to ensure collateral flow in alternate artery and within the palmar arch
Common and external iliac artery	1. Repair	
Common and external iliac vein	1. Repair	2. Can ligate
Femoral artery	1. Repair	
Femoral vein	1. Repair	2. Can ligate
Popliteal artery	1. Repair	
Popliteal vein	1. Repair	**Cannot ligate**
Tibial arteries	1. Repair	2. Can ligate but need to ensure patency of other distal arteries to foot

proximal and distal ends to achieve as much distance as possible. Having the entire extremity prepped into the sterile field allows manipulation of the limb to assess the level of tension intraoperatively.

When an appropriate vein conduit is unavailable, polytetrafluoroethylene (PTFE) grafts can be used. However, PTFE is associated with overall decreased patency rates and increased risk of thrombosis and infection in comparison to vein grafts. Intraluminal shunts using various conduits can be used to reperfuse the injured limb in unstable patients until definitive repair can take place.

If severe damage to the artery has occurred and adequate collateral circulation is available, ligation can be performed in certain arteries (see Table 17.3). Always attempt to guarantee patent flow in the collateral prior to ligation.

A post-repair arteriogram should be performed before leaving the OR to assess distal runoff after the repair. An exception to this may be in patients with an easily palpable distal pulse after completion of the repair (especially true in upper extremity reconstructions). Four-compartment lower extremity fasciotomies should also be done for repairs in the leg, especially in hemodynamically unstable patients, in patients with combined arterial and venous wounds, and in those with long ischemic times. Forearm and thigh fasciotomies can be indicated with certain injuries. It is important to realize that the distal muscle beds may not feel tight after repair. This is typical immediately after repair. Since the vascular injury and subsequent repair cause an ischemia-reperfusion injury to the distal muscle beds, the muscles may not swell initially from the reperfusion injury, but they ultimately will, causing a compartment syndrome. In the leg, the anterior compartment is the most susceptible to ischemia, and the deep posterior compartment is the one most frequently missed. Care must be taken to ensure adequate decompression of all four compartments.

Basic Operative Principles for Venous Injuries

In general, the basic tenets of arterial repair can be applied to venous injuries. Lateral venorrhaphy is the preferred method of venous repair. Ligation is another viable option in the extremities except for the popliteal vein – it cannot be ligated (see Table 17.3) due to the high rate of amputation following vein ligation. Saphenous vein interposition grafts have poorer outcomes in comparison to their use in arterial injuries but can be an option. Four-compartment fasciotomies are recommended to reduce the possibility of compartment syndrome in the lower extremity.

Upper Extremity Exposures and Repair

Vascular repair in the upper limb requires mastery of several exposures. From proximal to distal, these include gaining access to the axillary, brachial, radial, and ulnar vessels. Options for repair are included in each specific section below.

Axillary Artery and Vein

The origin of the axillary artery is at the lateral border of the first rib and extends to the lower margin of the teres major muscle, after which it becomes the brachial artery. The axillary artery has six branches and is divided into three parts, which are based on the relation to the pectoralis minor muscle:

- First part: above pectoralis minor
- Second part: deep to the pectoralis minor
- Third part: below the pectoralis minor

The axillary artery is surrounded by the brachial plexus, and the axillary vein lies medial to the artery; due to the proximity of these structures, corresponding vein and nerve injuries are often encountered.

Access to the axillary vessels is best approached through a transverse infraclavicular incision. Dissection is carried down through the pectoralis major muscle to the pectoralis minor muscle. The pectoralis minor tendon may be divided from the coracoid process, and the muscle retracted if exposure in this area is needed. The axillary vessels lie deep to the pectoralis minor.

Obtain proximal and distal control of the injured vessel, and then perform primary repair or resection and primary anastomosis if possible. Be sure to prep and drape the entire chest, shoulder, and arm. Abduction and adduction of the arm during surgery will allow a thorough assessment as to whether an interposition graft is necessary. If a graft is necessary, use the saphenous vein.

Brachial Artery and Vein

The brachial artery extends from the lower margin of the teres major to the antecubital fossa. The brachial vein and median nerve lie medial to the artery. The basilic vein and ulnar artery are more medial and superficial to the artery. The radial nerve is lateral, on the opposite side of the humerus.

Exposure of the brachial vessels is achieved with a longitudinal incision along the medial aspect of the upper arm between the biceps and triceps muscles. Simple arterial injuries can be repaired primarily. If the vessel is transected or if there is extensive loss of arterial length, a saphenous vein interposition graft is preferred. The brachial vein can be ligated. Consider forearm fasciotomies based on intraoperative swelling and compartment pressures.

Radial and Ulnar Arteries

The radial and ulnar arteries are the terminal branches of the brachial artery and supply the hand via the superficial and deep palmar arches. Injuries to the radial or ulnar arteries should raise suspicion of associated radial and ulnar nerve injuries, as each nerve courses the length of the forearm with the artery.

Proximal exposure of the radial and ulnar arteries can be achieved with an S-shaped incision across the antecubital fossa. Distal to the antecubital fossa, make a longitudinal incision over the artery. In cases of stab or cut-type injuries to the forearm, it may be feasible to extend the existing laceration. Primary repair of the arteries can be attempted but long-term patency rates are poor. Ligation of either artery can be done if an Allen's test is performed to guarantee collateral flow in the other artery, as well as sufficient blood flow in the palmar arch with the vessel clamped. Venous injuries in the forearm can be ligated with little consequence.

Lower Extremity Exposures and Repair

Lower extremity vascular trauma commonly occurs secondary to penetrating trauma, although certain blunt mechanisms result in fractures with specific vascular injuries (see Table 17.1). Gaining access and repairing femoral, popliteal, anterior tibial, posterior tibial, and peroneal artery injuries are an important skill set for the trauma surgeon.

Common and Superficial Femoral Artery

The common femoral artery is a continuation of the external iliac artery and begins at the inguinal ligament. It gives off the profunda femoris artery and becomes the superficial femoral artery as it descends toward the knee. The femoral triangle contains the femoral vein, artery, and nerve (medial to lateral) and is bound superiorly by the inguinal ligament, medially by the medial border of the adductor longus muscle, and laterally by the medial border of the sartorius muscle.

Exposure to control bleeding proximal to the common femoral artery requires either a retroperitoneal approach with an incision in the flank or a laparotomy to access the external iliac artery. To access the common femoral artery, a longitudinal incision can be made over the vessels distal to the inguinal ligament. The approach to the superficial femoral artery involves making an incision along the anterior border of the sartorius muscle. All arterial injuries should undergo repair, either primary with resection and anastomosis with appropriate mobilization or with an interposition saphenous vein graft from the contralateral thigh. Repair of the femoral vein should be attempted, but ligation is a secondary option. Four-compartment fasciotomies are recommended for arterial injuries and femoral vein ligation; a completion arteriogram for arterial injuries is also recommended.

Popliteal Artery and Distal Arteries

The popliteal artery is a continuation of the superficial femoral artery and begins at the adductor hiatus. It is the deepest structure in the popliteal fossa and is fixed proximally at the adductor hiatus and distally at the soleus insertion. This fixation makes it vulnerable to injury in blunt trauma, especially following posterior knee dislocation or proximal tibia fractures. The popliteal vein crosses the artery as it ascends through the popliteal fossa and is lateral above the knee.

The popliteal artery is best exposed through a medial incision above the knee. Division of the medial head of the gastrocnemius muscle will improve distal exposure, and division of the semimembranosus and semitendinosus muscles can improve proximal exposure. Primary repair is rarely possible. Repair is best achieved with a femoral-popliteal bypass using a reverse saphenous vein graft from the contralateral leg. PTFE grafts should be avoided at all costs. We typically inject tPA distally at the completion of the repair. Similarly, injuries in the anterior tibial, posterior tibial, and peroneal arteries are generally not amenable to primary repair. Ligation can be performed in these distal vessels if there is patent flow in the remaining distal vessels supplying the foot. If there is any doubt about collateral flow, an intraoperative arteriogram should be performed. Interposition grafts can be utilized as well in these distal vessels but are technically demanding.

Postoperative Care

In the immediate postoperative period, it is critical to monitor the vascular and neurologic exams routinely (e.g., every hour) and note any changes. Special attention should be paid to the pulse exam, any changes in motor or sensory function, compartment pressures (if prophylactic fasciotomies were not done), condition of muscle after fasciotomies, the patient's overall hemodynamic status, and any signs of infection or rhabdomyolysis. Any change in the vascular exam or signs of compartment syndrome necessitate immediate return to the operating room.

Take-Home Points
1. Control of hemorrhage with direct pressure or a tourniquet is the initial management of choice for extremity bleeding.
2. Hard signs of arterial injury include active hemorrhage, absent distal pulses, an expanding or pulsatile hematoma, a palpable thrill or bruit, and the five Ps (pain, pallor, paralysis, paresthesias, and poikilothermia).
3. After a vascular and neurologic exam, the next step in management of ongoing extremity hemorrhage is exploration and repair in the operating room.
4. Numerous operative strategies exist to repair injured vessels, including primary repair, resection and primary anastomosis, interposition grafts, shunts, and ligation.
5. Certain vascular injuries should be suspected with specific orthopedic injuries.
6. While repair of any injured vessel is generally preferred, some vessels, depending on location and collateral flow, can be ligated.

You can bleed as rapidly from 5 small blood vessels as you can from 1 large one. Harlan Stone

Suggested Readings

Magnotti L, Sharpe J, Fabian T. Peripheral vascular injuries. In: Peitzman A, et al., editors. The trauma manual: trauma and acute care surgery. 4th ed. Philadelphia: Woltzers Kluwer; 2013.
Sise J, Shackford S. Peripheral vascular injury. In: Mattox K, et al., editors. Trauma. 7th ed. New York: McGraw Hill; 2013.

Chapter 18
Endoscopic Hemorrhage: This is Even Harder than the Laparoscope!

Rachid Mohamed

Case Scenario

A 62-year-old obese, diabetic, cirrhotic patient with COPD and coronary artery disease has a massive upper gastrointestinal bleed. He is intermittently stable with resuscitation, and you identify a large bleeding duodenal ulcer on your endoscopy.

As an endoscopist, there are few instances more anxiety provoking and, at the same time, potentially satisfying as an acute gastrointestinal bleed. These clinical situations require prompt identification and intervention to ensure the highest likelihood of a positive outcome. Acute non-variceal upper gastrointestinal bleeding (UGIB), which is the focus of this chapter, remains a common medical condition with measurable mortality and morbidity. The annual incidence is between 50 and 150 cases per 100,000 adults [1].

Peptic ulcer disease remains the most common cause of non-variceal UGIB, accounting for 1/3 to 2/3 of cases [1]. Other causes of UGIB include mucosal erosive disease, such as esophagitis (7–31%), malignancy (2–8%), and Mallory-Weiss tears (4–8%). Less common etiologies include Dieulafoy lesions (submucosal arterioles), gastric antral vascular ectasia (GAVE), and an aortic-enteric fistula.

Initial Assessment and Resuscitation

Managing these patients starts well before the endoscopy suite. The clinical presentation of patients is highly dependent on the site of bleeding, etiology, and rate of blood loss. Visible bleeding can be seen in the form of emesis or passage of blood in the stool. Hematemesis can be bright red (indicating a more brisk or acute bleed)

R. Mohamed (✉)
Therapeutic Endoscopy, Peter Lougheed Centre, Calgary, AB, Canada
e-mail: rmmohame@ucalgary.ca

© Springer International Publishing AG 2018
C.G. Ball, E. Dixon (eds.), *Treatment of Ongoing Hemorrhage*,
DOI 10.1007/978-3-319-63495-1_18

Fig. 18.1 Peripheral intravenous access

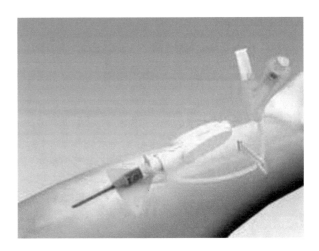

Fig. 18.2 Central intravenous access

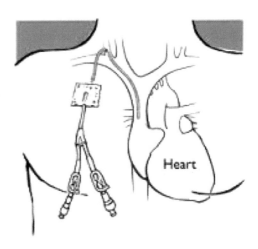

or coffee ground in color (indicating blood that has been in the stomach and altered by gastric acid). Similarly, blood in the stool can be fresh (bright red) or old (melena/black) with the former often an indicator of potential instability. Of course, blood in the stool is not exclusively an indicator of upper gastrointestinal bleeding and can be related to mid- or lower bowel bleeding sources.

Once a diagnosis of upper GI bleeding is established, fluid resuscitation is the first, and often the most important, step in management. Appropriate IV access, most often in the form of two large-bore (18-guage minimum) peripherally placed catheters, should be attained. In instances where there is peripheral shutdown of vasculature, central venous or intraosseous accesses are other options. All patients should be administered a bolus (1–2 L) of crystalloid solution (normal saline or lactated Ringer's) to correct immediate hypovolemia. Thereafter ongoing support of volume state and hemodynamics can be done by infusions of crystalloid solutions (Figs. 18.1, 18.2 and 18.3).

Fig. 18.3 Intraosseous intravenous access

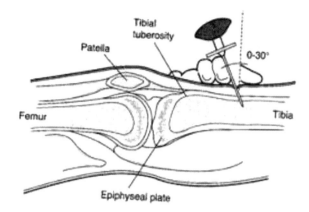

Transfusion requirements

- Transfuse red blood cells only if hemoglobin <70g/L, unless symptoms of anemia or significant cardiac disease
- Transfuse platelets only if platelet count <50 x 10^9/L or <100 x 10^9/L with suspected platelet dysfunction

Fig. 18.4 Transfusion requirements

All patients with acute UGIB should be typed and crossmatched for blood products. While transfusion of red blood cells can be life-saving in situations of severe hemodynamic compromise of active coronary artery disease, less aggressive transfusion strategies are preferred in most cases [2]. Overtransfusion can rapidly increase intravascular volume and result in further bleeding. In patients with a hemoglobin less than 70 g/L, the target hemoglobin for transfusion resuscitation is 70–90 g/L, and this more restrictive approach has been associated with less rebleeding and lower mortality [3]. The use of platelet transfusion is similarly restricted to severe thrombocytopenia [4] (Fig. 18.4).

Nasogastric Lavage

What was once a traditional dogmatic mainstay in the management of acute UGIB has largely fallen out of favor as a routine intervention [4]. The placement of a nasogastric (NG) tube is uncomfortable and not associated with any reduction in rebleeding or mortality [5]. There are rare instances where aggressive lavage through an oral gastric lavage system may be used to improve visualization, but routine placement of an NG tube is no longer advised.

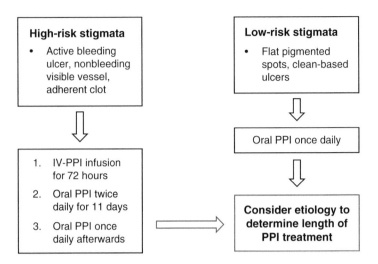

Fig. 18.5 Algorithm for proton pump inhibitor therapy for peptic ulcers based on endoscopic findings

Medical Therapy in Non-variceal UGIB

Often endoscopic visualization and delivery of necessary therapy is limited and hampered by the presence of blood and clots in the upper GI tract. The use of a prokinetic agent such as erythromycin 30 min prior to the planned endoscopy can help to clear contents from the upper GI tract. This intervention has been shown to shorten the duration of endoscopy and reduce the need for repeat endoscopy [6].

There has been controversy as to the merits (or lack thereof) of pre-endoscopic use of proton pump inhibitor (PPI) therapy. The largest meta-analysis on this issue, involving more than 2000 patients, concluded that pre-endoscopic proton pump inhibition therapy essentially downstages high-risk endoscopic lesions [7]. There were less patients with high-risk endoscopic lesions in the PPI-treated group and consequently less need for endoscopic intervention. When used, a bolus dose of 80 mg intravenously of PPI is administered followed by an infusion of 8 mg/hr. This infusion is continued until endoscopic intervention for diagnosis of the bleeding etiology. If endoscopy shows a low-risk lesion, the intravenous infusion of PPI can be discontinued and replaced by oral once-daily PPI therapy.

If endoscopic therapy is applied to an upper GI bleed, the intravenous PPI infusion is continued, although debate exists as to the duration. The premise is that acid suppressive therapy will increase clot stability and lessen the effects of acid on coagulation factors [4]. Evidence supports the continuation of IV PPI infusion for high-risk upper GI bleeding lesion that have been treated with endoscopic hemostasis measures [8]. Thereafter, the intravenous PPI therapy can be switched to oral. A reasonable approach to the use of proton pump inhibitor therapy in acute UGIB is shown below [4] (Fig. 18.5).

Helicobacter pylori Eradication

Helicobacter pylori (*H. pylori*) is an established contributing cause to upper GI bleeding. All patients presenting with an acute UGIB should be tested for *H.pylori* [9]. Serology is the preferred method as endoscopic biopsies or urea breath testing can be falsely negative during acute bleeding. If testing is negative during the acute incident, follow-up testing 4 weeks later should be undertaken to ensure a true negative status. Numerous antibiotic/PPI regimens exist and are largely determined by regional antimicrobial resistance patterns. Confirmation of eradication should be performed with a urea breath test.

Endoscopic Evaluation in Non-variceal UGIB

Peptic Ulcer Disease

Prompt endoscopic investigation and, at times, intervention is a critical component in the management of upper gastrointestinal bleeding. The risk of rebleeding of ulcerated lesions in the upper GI tract is related to the findings seen at the time of endoscopy (Forrest classification). Actively bleeding lesions (types Ia and Ib) have significant risks of rebleeding (approximately 40–55%) without endoscopic therapy [9]. Conversely, low-risk lesions such as clean-based ulcers or those with pigmented spots have a low risk of rebleeding (<10%) and often do not require endoscopic intervention. Utilizing this classification permits appropriate delivery of endoscopic therapy and disposition planning for the patient. Individuals with low-risk ulcer lesion can often be discharged home with oral proton pump inhibitor therapy (Figs. 18.6 and 18.7).

There are several endoscopic therapy options available for the management of bleeding peptic ulcers. These include injection therapy of epinephrine, coaptive coagulation, mechanical clip application, and use of hemostatic agents. Evidence strongly supports *not* using epinephrine injection in isolation but rather coupling it with a second endoscopic measure for improved outcomes [9].

Submucosal injection therapy allows fast but temporary reduction of acute gastrointestinal bleeding. An injection catheter is passed down the working channel of the endoscope into the field of view of the endoscopist. The needle is oriented tangentially to the mucosa at an angle of 20–70°. The target is to inject around the ulcer lesion, often in four quadrants, to achieve tamponade of the feeding submucosal vessel (see image below). Panels 1 and 2 show injection around the ulcer base with delivery of the injectate into the submucosa. Panels 3 and 4 highlight the completion of four-quadrant injection to complete the tamponade effect (Fig. 18.8).

The mainstay of injection therapy is diluted (1:10,000) epinephrine. Several studies have shown that large-volume (greater than 13 cc) injection offers hemostatic benefit over small volume but may carry potential risk of arrhythmia and

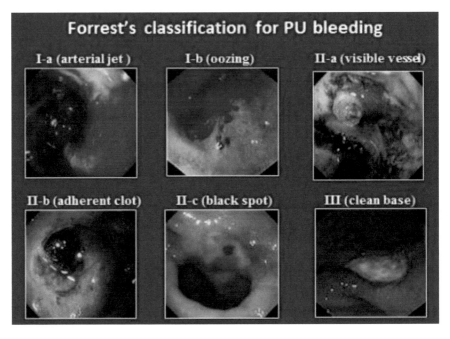

Fig. 18.6 Forrest's classification for PU bleeding

Endoscopic findings as predictors of clinical outcome

ENDOSCOPIC FINDING	PREVALENCE %	RECURRENT BLEEDING (%)	SURGERY (%)	MORTALITY (%)
Active bleeding	18	55	35	11
Visible vessel	17	43	34	11
Adherent clot	17	22	10	7
Flat spot	20	10	6	3
Clean-base ulcer	42	5	0.5	2

Fig. 18.7 Endoscopic findings as predictors of clinical outcome [26]

hypertensive crises [10–12]. The ideal injection solution remains to be clearly clarified. Some studies have shown similar bleeding outcomes with injection of distilled water or normal saline compared to epinephrine [13, 14]. This further highlights the notion that the main effect of submucosal injection is tamponade rather than vasoconstriction.

The delivery of coaptive coagulation is a well-established and widely used technique that is often coupled with submucosal injection. As mentioned above, dual endoscopic therapy (e.g., injection and thermal coagulation) is superior to injection monotherapy [15]. Thermal coagulation in the management of peptic ulcer disease strives to deliver coaptive coagulation. This entails mechanical pressure on the submucosal vessel to oppose the endothelial walls. Coagulation is then delivered to thermally seal the walls against one another and stop the blood flow. The thermal

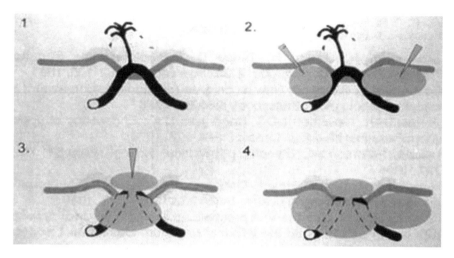

Fig. 18.8 Depiction of ulcer with submucosal blood vessel (panel **1**). Injection adjacent to ulcer (panel **2**) to achieve tamponade of feeding portions of the submucosal vessel. Injection into remaining quadrants around ulcer (panels **3** and **4**), complete injection therapy

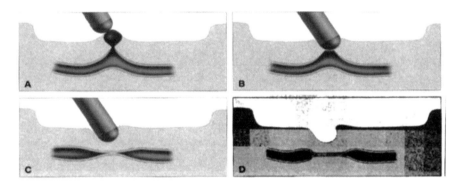

Fig. 18.9 (**a–d**) Coaptive coagulation

probe is passed down the working channel of the endoscope, and direct, firm pressure is applied to the base of the ulcer or visible vessel. Coagulation at 80 W is delivered through the probe while holding pressure on the ulcer base for 5–10 s. Water irrigation is then used to pull the probe off the ulcer base so as to limit sticking of the probe to the ulcer base. This can be repeated until a satisfactory result is achieved. Understandably, there is a risk of luminal perforation as the thermal coagulation is applied to the ulcer base [16]. This can be limited by direct endoscopic visualization of therapy application and limiting the force of pressure on the probe in the ulcer base (Fig. 18.9).

Mechanical closure of bleeding peptic ulcers is a highly effective modality that, unlike injection therapy, can be used as a monotherapy [15]. The premise is to apply mechanical closure of the visible vessel or feeding vessel for hemostasis.

Fig. 18.10 Mechanical
closure of visible vessel
with hemoclip

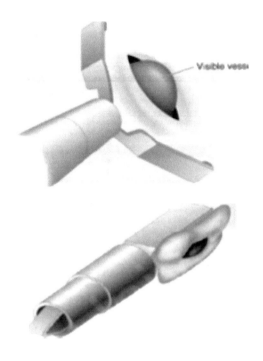

Numerous clip options are available with the main design consisting of opposing
surgical steel arms. The clip is passed in a closed format down the working channel
of the endoscope. The clip is then opened by the endoscopy assistant and can be
rotated (in most instances) into the ideal orientation, which is perpendicular to the
direction of the blood vessel. The clip is advanced against the vessel and closed
when the positioning is secured. Often, this will stop the bleeding instantly. The clip
is then deployed from the delivery device. Most endoclips remain in position for
3–14 days (Fig. 18.10).

An over-the-scope clip (OTSC) (Ovesco Endoscopy) is a novel tool that can be
used to manage large peptic ulcer bleeds [17]. This device, consisting of the clip
anchored on an endoscopic flexible plastic cap, is loaded on the tip of the endoscope
prior to insertion into the GI tract. Once the ulcer is visualized, an en face approach
is obtained. The ulcer base and surrounding tissue can be pulled into the cap using
different grasping tools and/or suction from the endoscope. Once the desired tissue
is in the cap, the clip is deployed via a rotating knob system outside the body. This
clip is felt to be more permanent as it grasps a larger amount of tissue than traditional endoclips.

The newest tool available for endoscopic management of acute non-variceal
upper GI bleeding is a hemostatic powder, called Hemospray (Cook Medical Inc.,
Winston-Salem, NC, USA). While the exact mechanism of action is not known, this
agent (along with others currently in development) is thought to increase the con-
centration of coagulation factors, activate platelets, and form a mechanical plug on
the injured vessel [18]. It was initially felt to be a salvage technique in refractory

Fig. 18.11 Image showing an actively bleeding gastric ulcer

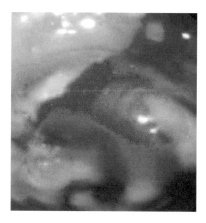

Fig. 18.12 Image showing appropriate positioning of Hemospray delivery catheter at an adequate distance from the bleeding ulcer

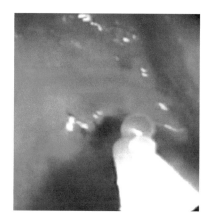

bleeding cases that have failed conventional methods of endoscopic hemostasis therapy. However, more and more, it is being used as an early intervention given its high efficacy and relative ease of use [19]. The delivery catheter is passed down the working channel of the endoscope. Care must be employed to have a dry working field, as any fluid will lead to the immediate coagulation of the powder. If this occurs prematurely, the delivery catheter can become occluded and will need to be replaced. Therefore, it is ideal to remain an adequate distance away from active bleeding, usually 3–5 cm. Once positioned, the powder is dispersed from the delivery catheter using a carbon dioxide propelling deployment system outside the body. The powder is dispersed in a wide field therefore making it relatively easy to target the bleeding site. The initial hemostasis results with Hemospray are quite promising, but more research into the robustness of this initial hemostatic effect and whether or not additional endoscopic therapies are required is still needed (Figs. 18.11, 18.12, 18.13 and 18.14).

Fig. 18.13 Deployment of
Hemospray powder

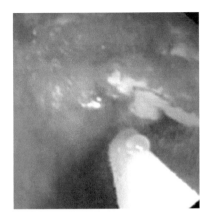

Fig. 18.14 Successful
hemostasis result on relook
endoscopy 24 h post
Hemospray

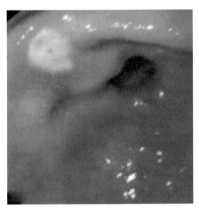

Other Causes of Upper GI Bleeding

Many of the therapeutic interventions (injection, cautery, clip application) translate over to other etiologies of upper GI bleeding. There are certain causes of bleeding that may require specific interventions.

Gastric Antral Vascular Ectasia (GAVE)

Visible columns of blood vessels radiating proximally from the pylorus characterize gastric antral vascular ectasia, also referred to as "watermelon stomach" [20]. This can present with overt or occult GI blood loss, with the latter often resulting in iron deficiency. The exact mechanism and pathophysiology are not understood, but it has been associated with a variety of medical ailments including cirrhosis, systemic sclerosis, diabetes mellitus, hypothyroidism, chronic renal failure, and cardiovascular disease.

Fig. 18.15 The targeted area is seen through the clear endoscopic cap on the end of the endoscope

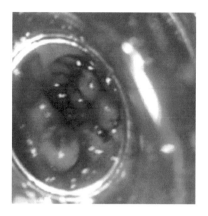

Fig. 18.16 Several bands are applied in a single endoscopic session

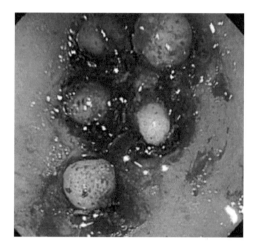

On endoscopic assessment of GAVE, generalized oozing from the gastric antrum is noted with often no primary or dominant bleeding site. As a result and given the diffuse nature of the condition, therapy is targeted to the entire affected region.

Endoscopic band ligation (EBL) involves the application of a rubber band to the mucosa/submucosa in an effort to strangulate feeding vasculature to the gastric antrum [20]. This is the same premise and involves the same endoscopic equipment, as for the treatment of esophageal variceal disease. The endoscopic band apparatus is loaded onto the endoscope prior to insertion into the body. On the end of the gastroscope is a clear, flexible cap. This cap is pressed perpendicularly to the targeted area, and the mucosa/submucosa is pulled into the cap using the suction function of the gastroscope. Once the tissue is entrapped in the cap, a single band is deployed using a handle outside the body. This can be repeated moving proximally from the pylorus with the end result being several bands applied in a single session (Figs. 18.15, 18.16 and 18.17).

Fig. 18.17 Follow-up
endoscopy showing
significant improvement in
GAVE

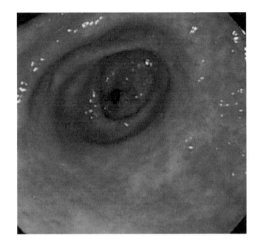

Fig. 18.18 Linear strips of
superficial antral vascular
change in GAVE is shown

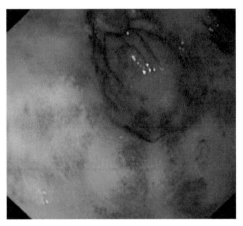

Coagulation of the superficial aberrant vasculature in GAVE is another effective endoscopic therapy option. Argon plasma coagulation (APC) involves the superficial cauterization of the targeted mucosa. The process involves the insufflation of argon gas through a probe that has been passed down the working channel of the endoscope. The probe is held a few millimeters above the mucosa, as this is a noncontact cautery therapy (as opposed to that used in the treatment of peptic ulcer disease). This probe then delivers an electric charge (50–70 W) through the control of the endoscopist. The result is the transmission of this electric charge through the argon gas medium to the mucosa [21]. Superficial cauterization of the mucosa is achieved with little to no energy delivery to deeper layers of the gastric tract. This method can be used to treat the affected are of GAVE in a "painting fashion" with complete treatment achievable in a single session [21, 22]. APC therapy is highly effective and repeatable option in the management of GAVE (Figs. 18.18, 18.19 and 18.20).

Fig. 18.19 Argon plasma coagulation is delivered to the targeted area

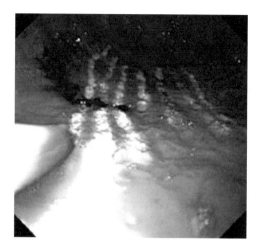

Fig. 18.20 End result showing extensive coagulation delivered to affected area

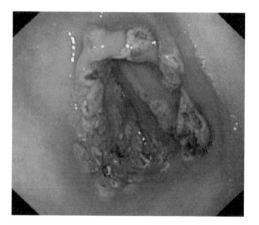

Dieulafoy's Lesion

Dieulafoy's lesion represents an uncommon but potentially serious etiology of upper GI bleeding. It involves an aberrant submucosal artery that erodes through the mucosa [23]. As an arterial source, the bleeding can be quite brisk and profound. The hallmark endoscopic finding is that of an active bleeding source, often within the gastric body, without surrounding mucosal ulceration to suggest peptic ulcer disease (Figs. 18.21 and 18.22).

The management of Dieulafoy lesions can prove challenging. These lesions are known to spontaneously retract back into the submucosa after an initial bleed. This results in difficulty identifying the source of bleeding during endoscopy. When the source is visualized, the arterial nature of the lesion often makes achieving hemostasis more difficult. A combination of the techniques described previously (injection,

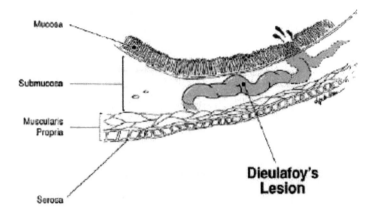

Fig. 18.21 Dieulafoy lesion with large penetrating submucosal vessel in the absence of mucosal ulceration

Fig. 18.22 Actively bleeding Dieulafoy lesion in the proximal stomach

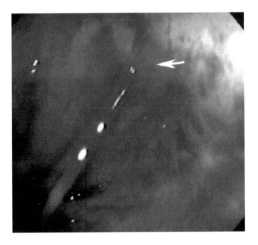

thermal, mechanical closure, and band ligation) is utilized. As a result of these factors, a small proportion of these lesions will require interventional angiography and targeting coiling of the lesion [23].

Mallory-Weiss Tear

Mallory-Weiss tear (MWT) is a laceration, often induced by vomiting, at the gastro-esophageal junction and a recognized cause of acute upper GI bleeding [24]. The majority of these cases will resolve with conservative measures such as time, fasting, and antiemetics. In cases where endoscopic intervention is required, mechanical closure with a hemoclip is most often utilized although studies have shown

Fig. 18.23 Actively bleeding Mallory-Weiss tear at the gastroesophageal junction

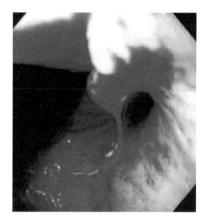

Fig. 18.24 Hemostasis post epinephrine injection therapy

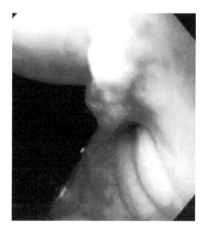

similar outcomes with injection therapy, cautery, and band ligation [25]. No repeat endoscopy is necessary once hemostasis is achieved, as the mucosal defect will heal on its own. In refractory cases, angiographic embolization can be employed (Figs. 18.23 and 18.24).

Take-Home Points
1. Gastrointestinal bleeding is a common problem with measurable morbidity and mortality
2. Appropriate identification and resuscitation is a critical first step in the management of non-variceal upper GI bleeding.
3. A conservative blood transfusion approach is favored.
4. Proton pump inhibitors do not influence mortality, surgery, or rebleeding but can help to downstage high-risk lesions at endoscopy.
5. Combination therapy is superior to injection therapy alone for the endoscopic management of peptic ulcer disease.

6. Mechanical closure is an equivalent hemostatic intervention to combination injection and coagulation therapy.
7. Novel hemostatic therapies, such as Hemospray, have high efficacy, but future research is required to assess the robustness of this intervention.
8. Causes of non-variceal UGIB other than peptic ulcer disease are less common and are highly treatable.

It is the most gratifying sign of the rapid progress of our time and technique that our best textbooks become antiquated so quickly. Theodor Billroth

References

1. Simon TG, Travis AC, Saltzman JR. Initial assessment and resuscitation in nonvariceal upper gastrointestinal bleeding. Gastrointest Endosc Clin N Am. 2015;25(3):429–42.
2. Meltzer AC, Klein JC. Upper gastrointestinal bleeding: patient presentation, risk stratification, and early management. Gastroenterol Clin N Am. 2014;43(4):665–75.
3. Villanueva C, Colomo A, Bosch A, et al. Transfusion strategies for acute upper gastrointestinal bleeding. N Engl J Med. 2013;368(1):11–21.
4. Fortinsky KJ, Bardou M, Barkun AN. Role of medical therapy for nonvariceal upper gastrointestinal bleeding. Gastrointest Endosc Clin N Am. 2015;25(3):463–78.
5. Huang ES, Karsan S, Kanwal F, et al. Impact of nasogastric lavage on outcomes in acute GI bleeding. Gastrointest Endosc. 2011;74:971–80.
6. Javad Ehsani Ardakani M, Zare E, Basiri M, et al. Erythromycin decreases the time and improves the quality of EGD in patients with acute upper GI bleeding. Gastroenterol Hepatol Bed Bench. 2013;6:195–201.
7. Sreedharan A, Martin J, Leontiadis GI, et al. Proton pump inhibitor treatment initiated prior to endoscopic diagnosis in upper gastrointestinal bleeding. Cochrane Database Syst Rev. 2010;7:CD005415.
8. Leontiadis GI, Sharma VK, Howden CW. Proton pump inhibitor therapy for peptic ulcer bleeding: Cochrane collaboration meta-analysis of randomized controlled trials. Mayo Clin Proc. 2007;82:286–96.
9. Barkun AN, Bardou M, Kuipers EJ, et al. International consensus recommendations on the management of patients with nonvariceal upper gastrointestinal bleeding. Ann Intern Med. 2010;152:101–13.
10. Park CH, Lee SJ, Park JH, et al. Optimal injection volume of epinephrine for endoscopic prevention of recurrent peptic ulcer bleeding. Gastrointest Endosc. 2004;60:875–80.
11. Lin HJ, Hsieh YH, Tseng GY, et al. A prospective randomized trial of large- versus small-volume endoscopic injection of epinephrine for peptic ulcer bleeding. Gastrointest Endosc. 2002;55:615–9.
12. Sung JY, Chung SCS, Low JM, et al. Systemic absorption of epinephrine after endoscopic submucosal injection in patients with bleeding peptic ulcers. Gastrointest Endosc. 1993;39:20–2.
13. Lai KH, Peng SN, Guo WS, et al. Endoscopic injection for the treatment of bleeding ulcers: local tamponade or drug effects? Endoscopy. 1994;26:338–41.
14. Lin HJ, Perng CL, Lee FY. Endoscopic injection for the arrest of peptic ulcer hemorrhage: final results of a prospective, randomized comparative trial. Gastrointest Endosc. 1993;39:15–9.
15. Marmo R, Rotondano G, Piscopo R, et al. Dual therapy versus monotherapy in the endoscopic treatment of high-risk bleeding ulcers: a meta-analysis of controlled trials. Am J Gastroenterol. 2007;102(2):279–89.

16. Chung SC, Leung JW, Sung JY, et al. Injection or heat probe for bleeding ulcer. Gastroenterology. 1991;100:33–7.
17. Park T, Wassef W. Nonvariceal upper gastrointestinal bleeding. Curr Opin Gastroenterol. 2014;30(6):603–8.
18. Changela K, Papafragkakis H, Ofori, et al. Hemostatic spray powder: a new method for managing gastrointestinal bleeding. Therap Adv Gastroenterol. 2015;8(3):125–35.
19. Babiuc RD, Purcarea M, Sadagurschi R, et al. Use of Hemospray in the treatment of patients with acute UGIB – short review. J Med Life. 2013;6(2):117–9.
20. Keohane J, Berro W, Harewood GC, et al. Band ligation of gastric antral vascular ectasia is a safe and effective endoscopic treatment. Dig Endosc. 2013;25(4):392–6.
21. Herrera S, Bordas JM, Llach J, et al. The beneficial effects of argon plasma coagulation in the management of different types of gastric vascular ectasia lesions in patients admitted for GI hemorrhage. Gastrointest Endosc. 2008;68(3):440–6.
22. Lecleire S, Ben-Soussan E, Antonietti M, et al. Bleeding gastric vascular ectasia treated by argon plasma coagulation: a comparison between patients with and without cirrhosis. Gastrointest Endosc. 2008;67(2):219–25.
23. Mumtaz R, Shaukat M, Ramirez FC. Outcomes of endoscopic treatment of gastroduodenal Dieulafoy's lesion with rubber band ligation and thermal/injection therapy. J Clin Gastroenterol. 2003;36(4):310–4.
24. Yin A, Li Y, Jiang Y, et al. Mallory-Weiss syndrome: clinical and endoscopic characteristics. Eur J Intern Med. 2012;23(4):e92–6.
25. Park CH, Min SW, Sohn YH, et al. A prospective, randomized trial of endoscopic band ligation vs. epinephrine injection for actively bleeding Mallory-Weiss syndrome. Gastrointest Endosc. 2004;60(1):22–7.
26. Laine L, Peterson WL. Bleeding peptic ulcer. N Engl J Med. 1994;331:717–27.

Chapter 19
Laparoscopic Hemorrhage: Do We Have to Open?

Scott Gmora

Case Scenario

You're performing a laparoscopic extended right hemicolectomy on a 72 year-old female for cancer when a little too much traction results in torrential venous haemorrhage from the right upper quadrant. The field turns red...

Many surgeons have found themselves trapped in this so-called laparoscopic snowball. It is a nightmare situation, the surgical equivalent of quicksand: the more you panic, the quicker you sink. Unless you have a clear plan of action in place before the case even begins, rest assured, you'll undoubtedly find yourself stuck in one of these snowballs at some point in your career. This chapter gives you a practical strategy for dealing with hemorrhage during laparoscopic cases.

Laparoscopy Is a Different Animal

Laparoscopy has clearly revolutionized the way we perform surgery. There's certainly been no shortage of papers regaling the virtues of minimally invasive surgery: everything from decreasing the length of hospital stays to reducing surgical site infections and postoperative pain.

The advent of specialized staplers, energy devices, and laparoscopic suturing techniques has allowed surgeons to push the surgical envelope further and further. Complex procedures that once seemed impossible to perform laparoscopically have become commonplace in the laparoscopic arena. Gastric bypass? Whipple procedure? AAA repair? Done, done, and done.

Scott Gmora, MD (✉)
General/Bariatric Surgery, St. Joseph's Healthcare, Mcmaster University,
Hamilton, ON, Canada
e-mail: gmora@mcmaster.ca

© Springer International Publishing AG 2018   233
C.G. Ball, E. Dixon (eds.), *Treatment of Ongoing Hemorrhage*,
DOI 10.1007/978-3-319-63495-1_19

With these advances, however, comes the realization that major surgical bleeding remains the great equalizer. If having to deal with serious bleeding during open surgery isn't harrowing enough, laparoscopic surgery serves to introduce a whole new level of pain to the game.

Developing Your Strategy Beforehand

The key to dealing with laparoscopic bleeding (or any bleeding, for that matter) is putting a well-developed strategy in place *before* you ever find yourself needing one in the first place.

Step 1: Initial Temporary Control

When you encounter a big (or potentially big) bleeder, your first move should almost always be to obtain initial *temporary* control. You have at your disposal a few precious seconds to see where the bleeding is coming from and to grasp or compress the vessel or surrounding tissue. If you miss this window, you'll quickly find that the accumulated blood has completely obscured the bleeding vessel—along with much of your visual field.

When faced with bleeding, I commonly see trainees of all levels frantically reach for their suction device or ask for a clip applier. *You need to resist this urge*. Often, by the time you've successfully introduced either of these instruments into the abdomen, your visual field will already have been lost, making it much more difficult to recover.[1]

If you can see the bleeding vessel, gently grasp it with an instrument in your nondominant hand. *A word of caution*: when grasping tissue, you always run the risk of turning a small side hole in a vessel into a major bleeder. If you can't see the vessel or feel it isn't safe to grasp (e.g., retracted vessel in the splenic hilum), you should instead consider compression with some radiopaque surgical gauze (e.g., Ray-Tec©).

Have you successfully brought the bleeding to a stop or at least to a slow trickle? If so, proceed *immediately* to Step 2. Do not readjust your hand to get a better grasp of the tissue. Don't start suctioning, and definitely don't start throwing clips everywhere. You have control; it's time to take a deep breath and regroup.

If you're unable to gain control of the bleeding, this is the point at which you'll need to start thinking about the possibility of having to convert to open. A good

---

[1] An exception to this rule is permissible when you see a small "pumper" with a clear pedicle or stalk. Sometimes, letting it bleed allows you to see the vessel more clearly, so that a clip can be easily applied.

surgeon will appreciate the gravity of the situation and will make the decision to open *before* the necessity of doing so becomes apparent to everyone around him or her. Don't wait for the patient to become hemodynamically unstable before making this decision. For a surgeon, there can be no greater tragedy than failing to convert to an open procedure as their patient exsanguinates right in front of them.

As soon as you become aware of the severity of the current situation, inform the scrub nurse that you may need to open, and ask him or her to prepare a 10 blade in the event that you do. There's nothing worse than trying to perform an emergent laparotomy with a tiny 15 blade normally used for trocar incisions.

Step 2: Stop What You're Doing!!!!!

This step is, without question, the most critical—and it's the key to dealing with any serious bleed you may encounter during laparoscopic surgery. What you do next will represent the difference between a small fender bender and ten-car pileup. Now that you have control, stop and regroup.

A. Calm Down

I realize that the worst thing you can tell someone who is panicking is to "calm down." The fact remains, though—in a situation as urgent as this—you *do* need to calm down. Your team is looking to you for leadership, your patient is relying upon you to save his or her life, and you're of no use to anyone if you can't first regain control of yourself.

Here are two of the best techniques I know for quickly snapping yourself out of a panic state:

1. *Consciously slow down your breathing.* Tons of research has been done in professional sports around the use of deep, diaphragmatic breathing as a tool to slow down one's heart rate and regain self-control. Once you have regained temporary control of the vessel, your next step should be to take a deep breath. You'll be amazed at how quickly this can bring you out of panic mode.[2]
2. *The "Mister Rogers Technique."* Ever notice that people who are panicking tend to raise their voices and speak really, really fast? Another great trick for quickly neutralizing panic is to deliberately lower the volume of your voice and speak more slowly—hence, the "Mister Rogers Technique." Consciously forcing yourself to speak like Mister Rogers ("Okay, boys and girls…") will instantaneously calm your mind and lower the chaos level in the room.

---

[2]An excellent book detailing the precise steps used by professional athletes to control their arousal state during competition is *10-Minute Toughness: The Mental Training Program for Winning Before the Game Begins* by Jason Selk. You'll be surprised at how much of the book directly applies to surgeons.

The next time you find that you have just ripped a hole in a major vessel, try simply grabbing the vessel, taking a deep breath, and, in your calmest voice, saying, "Hmmm...interesting." You'll look like a seasoned pro.

Step 3: Plan of Attack

Remember the laparoscopic snowball we discussed at the beginning of the chapter? This is where we do everything in our power to prevent it from ever launching down the mountain. As Benjamin Franklin famously said, "By failing to prepare, you are preparing to fail." This situation has now morphed into a game of simple strategy, and you should be thinking at least three moves ahead. The best way to ensure that your plan is smoothly executed is to run through a mental checklist prior to moving forward.

A. Equipment Checklist

1. You'll need at least one 12 mm (or larger) trocar in place (preferably for your dominant hand working port). If you don't have any in place, strongly consider upsizing one of the 5 mm ports now.
2. If the first rule of bleeding control in open surgery is to extend the incision, then the equivalent in laparoscopy is to add more trocars. Make sure there are extra trocars available and positioned close by, if needed (two 5 mm and one 12 mm trocar should suffice).
3. Ask the scrub nurse to open a package of 4 × 4-inch Ray-Tec© sponges (or any x-ray-detectable sponge).
4. Ensure that a clip applier is available and ready for use. If you are using a non-disposable clip applier, confirm that a clip is loaded and in place and that a sufficient number of other clips remain, if needed.
5. If you haven't already done so, ensure that an advanced energy-sealing device (ultrasonic, bipolar, etc.) has been opened and is ready to go.
6. Ask the nurse to test the suction device to ensure that it is working. Laparoscopic suction devices are notorious for getting clogged. If your assistant is inexperienced, consider disconnecting the irrigation tubing; there's a really good chance they will inadvertently douse the field with irrigant.
7. Make certain that your assistant/camera person has a trocar available to insert an instrument. It's ridiculous for the assistant to occupy his/her hands simply by holding the camera. This would be the equivalent of performing a laparotomy completely alone! Verify that there is a working port available for your assistant.
8. Do you need more hands? If so, now is the time to ask for additional help. Wait for your colleague(s) to arrive before attacking the belly of the beast.

9. Is the operative field properly exposed? If fat or other tissue keeps falling into the field, add another 5 mm port, and use a ratcheted grasper so an assistant can retract the problem away. Alternatively, place-change the patient's position to take advantage of gravity.
10. If there's a chance you'll need to quickly open, make sure that there's a 10 blade loaded on the scalpel handle.
11. For advanced laparoscopists, ensure that there's a laparoscopic needle driver loaded and ready to go.

B. Team Checklist

1. Inform the anesthesiologist that there is significant bleeding. It is critical that the patient not move at all during your attempt at hemostasis. If there is any question, strongly consider requesting that they administer additional paralytics.
2. Now is not the time for any of your team members to leave the room. Instruct the circulating nurse *not* to leave the room without first informing you.
3. *Do not* yell at or demean your assistant/camera person (regardless of how incompetent they may or may not be). This will only cause them to become more nervous and make more mistakes. There will be plenty of time for "constructive criticism" once you've regained control of the situation and have stopped the bleeding. Instead, provide specific guidance about how to avoid common pitfalls. You may say something like this:

We'll need to work together closely for this part of the case. Once the camera is in place, try your best not to move it around very much. Pay close attention to surrounding structures, and do your best not to accidentally smudge the camera lens on tissue or allow it to get hit by blood. If the camera lens becomes smudged or sprayed with blood, DO NOT remove the camera from the patient for cleaning unless I expressly instruct you to do so.

Step 4: Visualize and Recognize Anatomy

It goes without saying that blindly and haphazardly, clipping or coagulating the tissue is a move of desperation and should be avoided at all costs.

As previously mentioned, you should already have temporary control. If you haven't been able to attain it and there's no obvious arterial bleeding, the best bet is usually to simply compress the tissue with a piece of surgical gauze and wait. Better yet, place an absorbable hemostatic agent (e.g., Surgicel©) beneath the gauze prior to compression so you won't pull off any clots when the sponge is later removed.

The goal here is to try to visualize the bleeding vessel as clearly as possible *without losing control of it*. This is the surgical equivalent of snake handling. You need to deftly wrangle the adjacent tissue back and forth between your graspers, inching closer and closer to the culprit vessel until control is achieved. Your assistant should have a suction device in a place to help evacuate any blood that accumulates, allowing your surgical field to remain unobscured.

Step 5: Definitive Hemostasis

Never attempt definitive control of bleeding without knowing what your *next* move will be if the first attempt fails. If you are successful at gaining initial temporary control, resist the urge to impulsively go straight for definitive hemostasis (e.g., taking a wild bite with your energy device, blind clipping, etc.). The best strategy is to assume that your attempt at hemostasis *will* fail and to anticipate *in advance* what you will do, should this prove to be the case.

Many instances of severe bleeding will begin as a small herald bleed. For example, you might be taking the short gastrics during a fundoplication when you notice mild bleeding around the jaws of your energy device as you come across the tissue. The mistake would be to impulsively attempt an imprecise *second* bite with your energy device; this invariably transforms that same mild bleeding into a spurting jet of blood. If the bleeding is mild or if you have obtained temporary control, it's time to put together a cohesive plan of attack.

If the visualized culprit vessel is inessential to the patient's survival or to the integrity of the current surgical case, don't hesitate to definitively sacrifice it using the myriad tools at your disposal:

1. Application of a simple Hem-o-lok© clip[3]
2. Use of an appropriate energy device (ultrasonic or bipolar)
3. Laparoscopic stapled transection with a vascular load (2.0–2.5 mm)[4]

The appropriate choice of device depends on a host of factors, including your experience and comfort with the device in question, the size of the vessel, whether the vessel is partially or completely transected, the presence and length of the vascular pedicle, the proximity of adjacent viscera, and the projected degree of difficulty in regaining control if your initial attempt at definitive control fails.

If the culprit vessel cannot be sacrificed, then you have a bigger problem on your hands. If you are dealing with a sizeable hole, then some form of vascular suturing will likely be required. At this point, you'll need to look in the mirror and be brutally honest with yourself. Do you have the necessary laparoscopic skills to confidently load a needle on a driver, take precise bites of the vessel wall, and tie a proficient surgical knot? If your laparoscopic experience has been mainly limited to cholecystectomies, appendectomies, and hernias, *now is not the time to try your hand at advanced laparoscopic suturing.* Unless you suture laparoscopically on a very regular basis (simulators do not count!), I would strongly advise against attempting to do so in the middle of a serious bleed. There's simply no room for error, and even an

---

[3] While two clips on the proximal end are ideal, *they are not essential.* Do not risk adding a second clip if you feel that it would be technically challenging to do so. Your instinct is probably correct, and you don't want to risk rebleeding.

[4] A word of caution here: the ergonomics and use of laparoscopic vascular stapling devices require a surprisingly high level of experience and finesse. As is true with all laparoscopic devices, unless you have experience using the device, it would be really unwise to employ it now.

expert at laparoscopic suturing would find such a situation challenging (i.e., one-handed needle loading, dealing with suboptimal port placement, precise needle tip placement with imperfect visualization, etc.).

Making the Decision to Open

Even the most junior surgical resident knows that consideration should always be given to converting to a laparotomy whenever significant bleeding is encountered during a laparoscopic case. In reality, however, the decision is not always so obvious. It's surprisingly easy for surgeons to get trapped in a form of tunnel vision in which they lose sight of just how much bleeding has actually occurred (and how much time has elapsed) while they've been attempting to gain hemostatic control. While there's no magic cutoff point or sign that surgeons can reliably reference to trigger their decision to open, it would be wise to remember the following caveats:

1. Most surgeons wait far too long before opening. It takes a lot of guts to convert to a laparotomy after having worked diligently for hours to complete a case laparoscopically. A good surgeon, however, knows when to cut their losses. *No patient should EVER hemorrhage to death during a laparoscopic procedure.*
2. Here's a good rule of thumb: if the thought so much as enters your mind that you might need to open, you're probably right. Prepare for this possibility as soon as your instincts tell you that you've just poked the bear. Make sure that there's a large scalpel loaded, that a laparotomy case cart is in the room, and that the team knows that you may need to open at a moment's notice.

Specific Scenarios

Port-Site Bleeding

Clearly, the best way of dealing with port-site bleeding is to prevent it from occurring in the first place. If that ship has already sailed, you'll want to at least be able to identify the bleeding before the patient rolls out of the operating room (the majority of post-site bleeds are missed by surgeons at the time of surgery). Here are some general tips:

1. The "safest" location on the abdominal wall for trocar insertion is in the midline and/or lateral to the *linea semilunaris*.
2. If possible, use bladeless trocars, as they tend to cause less bleeding.
3. Transilluminate the abdominal wall to identify vessels prior to inserting your trocar.

4. Compulsively inspect the intraperitoneal trocar defects for at least 5 s after removing each trocar.

Managing Port-Site Bleeding

As with all bleeding, management of port-site bleeding begins with temporary control. This can generally be accomplished by either reinserting a trocar into the bleeding port site and applying torque or by using double-finger compression with your index finger placed through the peritoneal defect and with your thumb on the outside. Though rarely necessary, a Foley catheter can also prove effective. Use the largest catheter possible with a 30 ml balloon. Pull up and clamp in place with a hemostat.

Once you have gained temporary control, your attention can be turned to definitive hemostasis. Although you can extend the port skin incision as necessary, beware of chasing a bleeding epigastric vessel that has already retracted, as it is usually infective. For significant bleeding, the simplest and most effective technique tends to be a fascial closure device (e.g., Carter-Thomason© suture passer) with a figure-of-eight stitch.

Occasionally, one or more large transmural (from the outside in) nylon sutures on a long, curved needle may be necessary to obtain control in the case of retracted vessels. If this occurs, remember to remove the sutures early (i.e., within 24 h) to prevent full-thickness abdominal wall necrosis. Angiographic embolization is generally only considered in extremely unusual situations and as a last resort.

Vascular Injury on Initial Entry

There are few situations more harrowing than a major vascular injury on initial entry into the abdomen. While a discussion of proper laparoscopic entry techniques is beyond the scope of this chapter, suffice it to say that investing a few extra minutes to securing safe access can avert a serious disaster. Do not rush this part of the case!

When a major vascular injury occurs, one of two things will generally happen:

A. There will be uncontrolled free hemorrhage into the peritoneal cavity.

In this scenario, there is often complete red-out of the camera image immediately upon entry into the abdomen, or blood in the trocar itself. You have a few precious seconds to decide whether or not to rapidly convert to a laparotomy for vascular control. In this situation, the fatal error in judgment is failure to recognize the *possibility* of a major bleed and ignorantly spending an undue amount of time trying to repeatedly clean the camera lens or apply antifog while the patient bleeds out.

B. There will be retroperitoneal containment of the bleeding.

This situation is scary, because it is so easy to miss it entirely during the operation. Often, it only presents with fluid-responsive or -unresponsive hypotension in the PACU (see below).

Occasionally, this retroperitoneal blood will track to the upper abdomen and present with perihepatic or perisplenic bleeding/hematoma. So, if you see a moderate amount of unexplained blood around the liver and spleen upon initial entry, you'll need to definitively rule out the possibility of an occult retroperitoneal bleed.

Place the patient in reverse Trendelenburg, flip the greater omentum upward, and tuck it underneath the liver. Then, use both hands to sweep the entire small bowel to the upper abdomen. Carefully examine the retroperitoneum for a hematoma. With modern, high-quality camera optics, you may even be able to see the defect where the trocar pierced through the retroperitoneal fat.

Hypotension in the PACU

Postoperative hypotension indicates serious bleeding until proven otherwise. The majority of patients (though not all) with significant postoperative bleeding will present with fluid-responsive hypotension in the recovery room. The nurse anesthetist will invariably attribute the hypotension to the administration of narcotics. They will smile and tell you to relax and not to worry so much. *Do not listen to them*!!! They have little appreciation of the surgical procedure that has just been performed. Ensure adequate IV access, fluid resuscitate, and throw in a Foley catheter. If the patient's pressure does not respond or responds only transiently, you *must* return to the *or* to rule out bleeding. Delaying your decision until blood test results are available is a bad move, since hemoglobin almost always reads as normal this soon after a bleed and prior to resuscitation.

What if the patient is becoming progressively unstable and there's a genuine diagnostic dilemma (e.g., evidence of cardiac ischemia or pulmonary embolism) and/or there's no *or* available for immediate use? You can consider opening one of the 12 mm port sites in the recovery room (including the fascia stitch, if one has been placed). This is essentially a diagnostic peritoneal aspiration (DPA). If there's visible blood, hightail it back to the *or*.

Make the suggestions in this chapter a top priority during your laparoscopic cases, and you'll save yourself—and, more importantly, your patients—a lot of unnecessary grief.

Take-Home Points
1. Do not enter the abdomen until all of your equipment is properly set up and ready to go. Inserting a Veress needle before your camera or suction is hooked up is just plain dumb.
2. Ray-Tecs© are your friend. They only cost a few cents, and they can get you out of a jam in a pinch. Ask for them on all of your laparoscopic case carts.

3. If you see blood bubbling out from the jaws of your energy device as you come through tissue, take your finger off the button and *stop*. This may seem counter-intuitive—shouldn't you apply even more energy to thoroughly "cook" the tissue and stop the bleeding? The answer is *no*. When you see bleeding from the closed jaws of your energy device, it often indicates that you have only partially transected the vessel. If you continue coagulating, your vessel will retract, and it will become harder to control. Instead, stop coagulating, and suction to expose the bleeding vessel. Now you can take a second, larger bite across the entire width of the vessel.

4. Don't take your eyes off the monitor while you are being handed an instrument. Doing so is a rookie move.

5. If you ever get called from the floor regarding bleeding from a laparoscopic incision, think twice before simply placing a stitch to re-approximate the skin. You may very well find that you'll be called again an hour later, with bleeding coming from another incision. I've seen residents place sutures in three or four port sites before eventually realizing that the bleeding is actually originating intra-peritoneally and simply evacuating out of the ports. Don't get caught playing *surgical whack-a-mole*.

6. Occasionally, you can get yourself out of a jam by using a suture that contains a large clip at its free end. After you take a bite through the tissue with your needle, cinch down on the suture, and lock it into place with one or two additional clips. This is essentially a poor man's "LAPRA-TY®"—no need to throw a knot.

Operative atlases never bleed. Mosche Schein

Chapter 20
Hemorrhage in Prehospital and Extreme Environments: We Can't Just Go Home

Andrew W. Kirkpatrick

Case Scenario

You are a 23-year-old special forces operative deep behind enemy lines when you are involved in a firefight that injures one of your team members. He sustains a large-caliber gunshot wound to his left upper extremity. You are still engaged and under fire…

Critical Point: Stop the Bleeding! Stop the Bleeding! Stop the Bleeding!

Those are the first three things you should do to prevent unnecessary death before you can "relax" and breathe a slight sigh of relief when you move your live friend out of active gunfire or maybe a greater sigh if he/she survives to formal care facility, whereupon the relative resources, both human and infrastructure, will increase exponentially. That will be a spectacular success and greatly increase the chances that your basic training buddy, co-astronaut, or maybe even child will survive to enjoy a celebratory beer, Tang, or Shirley Temple upon the anniversary of their "survival." If the patient is yourself and you saved your own life with self-care, then we suggest all of the above. Stopping the bleeding is the most productive thing anybody can do for an injured person, and often simple interventions will suffice. It sounds simple, can be incredibly complex to the point of being elusive, but ultimately requires immediacy and the application of basics mostly involving your fingers, with some potential adjuncts. Many people who die unnecessarily could thus be saved, especially in cases of extremity hemorrhage. If the bleeding is intra-cavitary, however, there are fewer prehospital options. Rescuers should not

A.W. Kirkpatrick (✉)

Departments of Surgery and Critical Care Medicine, Foothills Hospital, Calgary, AB, Canada

e-mail: Andrew.kirkpatrick@albertahealthservices.ca

© Springer International Publishing AG 2018   243

C.G. Ball, E. Dixon (eds.), *Treatment of Ongoing Hemorrhage*,

DOI 10.1007/978-3-319-63495-1_20

underestimate human physiology and vitality, however, which may allow survival via hemostatic reflexes. Fluid resuscitation to raise blood pressure in a situation wherein the bleeding cannot be addressed is typically unwarranted. If hemorrhage control cannot be offered, at least responders should not undermine or sabotage human survival reflexes with misguided "non-therapeutics." Finally, there may be technically advanced intracavitary interventions to rescue the dying, but at present these are not "practical," except for consideration in research or exceptional operational situations.

Immediate Concerns

Your immediate concern is to "stop the bleeding" no matter what. Even if resuscitation fluids and/or blood products are available (which they probably aren't), shed blood can never be replaced without a penalty of heat loss, logistical input, and especially immune activation and toxic biomediator generation. Just as important is not to exacerbate the bleeding by (1) lack of action, (2) excessive observation, (3) or unwarranted resuscitation. So don't freeze, gawk, or overreact either. Implicit in this discussion is that you can "find the bleeding." If there is massive external hemorrhage, this will be obvious. However, intracavitary bleeding may be difficult to discern before the effects of massive blood loss are catastrophically apparent. Thus, massive intracavitary hemorrhage needs to be inferred from the location or mechanism of injury, and a high index of suspicion is warranted. Unfortunately this often directly conflicts with the requirement for mission completion in tactical or operational situations.

External Hemorrhage

If you see the blood, at least you know where to begin to stop the bleeding. The first intervention is to directly apply pressure, typically with a finger or hand. Wearing a glove is great if you have one, and universal precautions are "better," but if the victim is your team member, co-astronaut, child, or yourself, the risk of blood-borne diseases will likely be an irrelevant concern in the heat of the moment. If your fingers stop the bleeding, you have great options for simplifying your physical attachment to the patient. While simply holding a finger on the potential source of exsanguination may be very effective, you as a rescuer may need to drive the vehicle, return effective suppressive fire, or assess other casualties, etc., and thus, adjuncts to topical hemorrhage control may save the situation. In this regard, there has been a remarkable effort catalyzed by the necessities of the recent Near East conflicts to develop effective topical hemorrhage control agents that can be categorized into three broad categories of hemostatic bandages. These (1) concentrate clotting factors at the site of injury, (2) form a mucoadhesive barrier, or (3) actively activate the clotting cascade or supply exogenous clotting factors at the site of injury. To date none of these options have been conclusively proven superior to another, and practically all are likely better than your rolled up T-shirt. Realistically, the critical characteristics are the ability to conform to the wound geometry, be it a catastrophic multidimensional improvised explosive device wound, a gigantic blunt degloving, or a small penetrating wound. Therefore, if a hemostatic bandage is at hand, it should be firmly inserted into the wound physically compressing any cavity. If bleeding continues through the dressing, we recommend not removing and repeating the packing but more aggressively packing with additional dressing until the bleeding stops. Thereafter guidelines recommend supplementing the packing with an elastic-type pressure dressing overtop of the wound packing. We believe that a more expeditious solution for tactical and extreme environments would be to utilize a wound clamp to provide mechanical compression overtop of wound packing, a solution that has proven superiority in animal experiments and one that would minimize rescuer time and effort, by giving the responder back the full use of their hands as the wound clamp retains the packing rather than a need for manual pressure.

External Bleeding that Does NOT Digitally Occlude

If digital pressure does not stop the bleeding, there is a bigger problem, potentially *TREMENDOUS TROUBLE*. If the bleeding is from a limb, then the probable solution is the application of a tourniquet either by the victim (auto-application) or by a rescuer. A practical discretionary factor is whether the victim will be required to use the injured limb (self-extrication, defensive fire, etc.) as application of a tourniquet with effective arterial occlusion equates to complete sacrifice of limb function and ischemic pain that even the most motivated special forces or astronaut personality cannot ignore. Any caregivers who have never had an arterially occlusive tourniquet applied are strongly advised to try one, so they "understand."

The consistent adoption and dissemination of tourniquets' availability to all war fighters and their care providers have had a dramatic effect on reducing mortality from extremity wounds in the recent conflicts. Ideally every participant in a dangerous activity will have their own tourniquet and can ideally begin immediate hemorrhage control upon themselves assuming they have not lost consciousness, been paralyzed, or have more exsanguinating extremity wounds than tourniquets available (Fig. 20.1). If it is safe for responders to provide more than self-care, this is a better situation. Thus, if a victim can be provided care and simple compression does not immediately control the bleeding, a tourniquet should be placed to occlude the pulse in the affected extremity. In the case of an amputation or massively destructive wound, there is no limb function to consider, and proceeding directly to tourniquet is warranted. The end justifies the means, and as many tourniquets as it takes is appropriate to control the bleeding including multiple tourniquets on one limb. To be effective, tourniquets need to be clearly applied proximal to the site of bleeding.

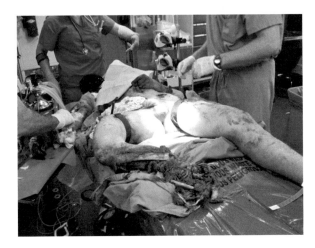

Fig. 20.1 Devastating extremity hemorrhage with exsanguination potential. Multiple injured extremities with loss of a responsible expectation that the victim can participate in any self care. Hemorrhage control should be provided through the early application of as many tourniquets as are required to control bleeding. Ultimately five tourniquets were applied to four limbs of this victim of an improvised explosive device in Afghanistan

In cases where the bleeding site is not obviously apparent and the environment does not lend itself to a careful examination, the Tactical Combat Casualty Care (TCCC) guidelines recommend placing the tourniquet "high and tight" on the injured limb to provide early effectiveness. If this is not effective, then a second tourniquet should be applied side by side with the first. While the goal of an effective tourniquet is occlusion of the arterial pulse, cessation of bleeding is more than an adequate goal in the early phases of care in hostile environments.

After tourniquets have been applied, every effort must be made to minimize the length of time of their application. If a tourniquet can be safely converted to a pressure dressing, wound packing, or wound clamp without bleeding resuming, then this is preferable. Thus, it is permissible to release a tourniquet that has been hastily applied in an emergency in a careful controlled manner if the victim is in a safe location. This allows evaluation of the wound. If the bleeding recommences, then the tourniquet should be immediately reapplied. This step is obviously unnecessary with massively destructive wounds or a complete amputation. If rebleeding necessitates reapplication of the tourniquet(s), then every effort is required to transport the patient to an operative facility with surgical capabilities for definitive therapy. In such cases it is important for all to recognize that there is potential limb compromise at the expense of saving life and that a patient who required an effective tourniquet to prevent exsanguination is not "stable" and should not be prioritized as such.

External Bleeding that Does NOT Digitally Occlude but Is NOT Amenable to Tourniquet

If digital pressure does not stop the bleeding and the wound is in one of the junctional regions of the body such as the groins, axillae, or neck, there is a very big problem, potentially *CATASTROPHIC TROUBLE*. The fundamental challenge is that tourniquets cannot be effectively applied in these challenging anatomic areas. In a care under fire setting, the best and potentially only option will be for the casualty or potential caregivers to move from the immediate danger zone to some cover as any intervention will be complex, time-consuming, and resource-consuming. Complex mechanical compressive devices either of the groin itself or the distal aorta are potentially available but require time, experience, and great mechanical pressure to be effective. Wound clamping is another option, that may even be self-applied, but does risk the simple conversion of external bleeding to internal bleeding with an expanding hematoma. Simplistically, any bleeding control is better than none. Potentially other increasingly elegant solutions are to pack the junctional wound with anything immediately available. From an optimistic perspective, the more hemostatic the packing, the better, but anything is better than nothing. The science tells us that holding pressure on this packed wound for 3 min is as effective as applying a wound clamp to contain the packing material. If the environment is hostile or other pressing tasks/duties/casualties require attention, then wound clamping may have an obvious advantage. An option that should never be forgotten if you have one is balloon catheter tamponade. If someone is exsanguinating, then inserting a balloon into the wound and inflating it may be lifesaving and permit safeextraction. In such cases this may be a bridge to definitive care, or it may be definitive if bleeding has ceased after 24 h when balloons are deflated in some experienced centers.

Once the casualty is removed from immediate danger and it is safe for caregivers to interact, it may be appropriate to bring remote portable point-of-care (POC) ultrasound to bear. Of all the technological medical advances of the last decade, ultrasound technology has been among the most disruptive in emergency care. Most if not all resuscitations now incorporate POC ultrasound, and this modality is increasingly likely to be in the hands of responders in prehospital and extreme environments. Thus, paramedical responders are increasingly being trained to utilize ultrasound in the field with or without real-time medical oversight. Thus, prehospital diagnoses of exsanguination into the pleural and peritoneal cavities should typically be recognized earlier, as should pericardial fluid, potentially directing transport, triage, and even interventions in prehospital environments. A more likely scenario with real-time telemedical/tele-ultrasound mentoring guidance is the actual detection of the bleeding site with Doppler-guided ultrasound and, once identified, evaluating the effective physical compression of this hemorrhage.

Bleeding that Does NOT Digitally Occlude Because It Is on the Inside

Realistically massive intracavitary hemorrhage in a tactical or extreme environment is probably going to be lethal, and all involved should share their last emotions freely and with as many tears as are appropriate. Thus, major noncompressible torso hemorrhage in prehospital environment of any kind is at best *TREMENDOUS TROUBLE* and not unlikely to be *CATASTROPHIC TROUBLE*. In a "simpler, safer" prehospital environment, the responders should simply "drive fast" as there are no helpful interventions in the prehospital arena for massive intracavitary hemorrhage. An unknown quandary concerns the issue of concomitant head injury as hypotension has been shown to generate far worse outcomes, yet prehospital fluid resuscitation in the fact on of ongoing hemorrhage propagates coagulopathies, continued bleeding, and inflammation. Thus, the prehospital solution may again be to simply "drive faster." In other words, gasoline is your most important resuscitation fluid.

Minimizing Internal Bleeding

While beyond the scope of this chapter, the hemostatic and homeostatic capabilities of the human body are simply stupendous and have all too often been discounted by physicians. It is remarkable how natural hemostasis will control massive bleeding especially after a period of hypotension (i.e., allowing initial clot stabilization). Thus, while the mechanism of action remains unknown, we do adhere to current guidelines concerning admission of tranexamic acid for prevention of hyperfibrinolysis. We also support the philosophy of not over-resuscitating with fluids. If a casualty is conscious or has a radial pulse, we do not initiate intravenous fluids. If any casualty does NOT have a radial pulse, we immediately respond with the recognition that patients in this subcategory possess a markedly increased risk of mortality. All should recognize that while profoundly important, hypotension is a poorly measured variable. While this is the single most important factor we use to guide activation responses, prehospital blood pressure measurement is an absolutely inexact science with 50% accuracy (akin to flipping a coin). Thus, if system efficiencies can be attained, more accurate prehospital identification of truly "sick" hypotensive patients is required, which may in the future involve POC lactate testing or various derivations of near-infrared spectroscopy.

Other tenants of minimizing internal bleeding involve (1) not mobilizing the casualty unless necessary as this will increase overall cardiac output, (2) not unnecessarily attempting to distract the bony pelvis, and (3) not delaying transport to an appropriate trauma center.

Specific Environments

Prehospital medicine, tactical medicine, extreme medicine, expedition medicine, and wilderness medicine can be considered as distinct specialties from an organizational and special interest viewpoint. They all share the same basic challenges; however, needing to balance possessing the most practically effective equipment to arrest potential hemorrhage when bringing anything imposes a liability to those bringing it. Extreme medicine can be defined as medicine practiced in any challenging or hostile physical environment. Expedition medicine specifically includes all facets of health care delivered in preparation for and during an expedition, typically in a remote geographical setting. Wilderness medicine is the unique body of knowledge that encompasses the basic science, physiology and pathophysiology, clinical practice, and research related to human interactions with the natural environment, as well as medicine practiced in remote locations or austere settings.

Prehospital

The primacy of simply attempting to stop external hemorrhage versus ignoring it as a determinant of grassroot survival recently received the US Presidential endorsement with the launch of a public service campaign entitled "Stop the Bleed." This initiative recognizes that otherwise potentially salvageable victims may exsanguinate before ANY trained responders arrives on scene. In nuts and bolts form, any hemorrhage control (presumably direct pressure or a tourniquet) is better than none and may be lifesaving. The featured techniques are tourniquet application and direct pressure. This should be considered an obligation of citizenship in any so-called developed country. More specifically, there is an obligation of one citizen to lay hands upon any other to "stop the bleed" when it occurs, without waiting for professionals to arrive after the citizen has exsanguinated. This is a particularly appropriate "responsibility" in societies with the "right" for citizens to freely arm themselves with massively destructive firearms.

Tactical Environments

Tactical medicine reflects medical care delivered in adverse environments where the risk of catastrophic additional wounds to both the patient and any responder is of concern. Often there will be NO possibility of another responder, thus mandating self-care for hemorrhage control as the only alternative. Many, if not most, of the simple principles of tactical medicine are derived from reflections within the US military and when introduced were seemingly at odds with civilian doctrine. However, even civilian thinking has progressed and validated these "military medicine" principles. Without reproducing the US military's TCCC recommendations, they can be summarized as basic common sense in a killing zone (where unfortunately you might not be able to think at all). If you find yourself in such a predicament, pure Darwinian forces will likely come to play based on the selected characteristics of clarity of thought under duress. If you are wounded somewhere and that humans, animals, or even aliens are still trying to kill you, you need to continue to fight back, or they will kill you. Hopefully you are armed in which case continue to use that weapon at all costs. If you are not armed or brought a knife to a gunfight, then you need to assess whether you are better running or hiding; recognizing the wrong decision will likely be fatal. To *allow* you to fight, run, or hide, you *should* control external hemorrhage on yourself if you can. But again, do not apply a completely immobilizing tourniquet on your dominant arm if this allows bad guys to walk up to you and kill you close range because you can't fire your weapon from ischemia within your arm.

What you are able to complete in terms of self-care will largely reflect what you have brought with you. This reality is typically defined by whether you are on a special forces mission or an unarmed civilian desperately trying not to be taken by kidnappers. If you have nothing but your skin and clothes, use your hand to compress the bleeding and thereafter any piece of clothing compressed and stuffed into the wound to "pack" the bleeding. In such a tactical setting, sterility is a luxury you cannot afford; you need to do anything and everything to *STOP THE BLEEDING*. If the wound is to an extremity, you can decide to apply a tourniquet. When effectively applied (occlude the pulse), this limb will become completely ischemic in 5–10 min and precluding running or climbing, respectively.

After critical evaluation of the Near East conflicts over the last several decades involving asymmetric warfare against nontraditional combatants and small-unit engagements (i.e., instead of the set piece battles of the last century), an array of sophisticated wound dressings with multiple characteristics have been advanced. In reality, none of these dressings have proven superior to the others, but the current TCCC guidelines recommend Combat Gauze as the hemostatic dressing of choice, followed by Celox Gauze or ChitoGauze. Clearly any choice is superior in your hand if an ambulance will never come. How you employ these dressings is more important than which one you choose. However, it is critical to stuff the bandage within the wound rather than just place it on the site. If you have a self-adherent wound clamp, it will also hold the dressing in place to occlude hemorrhage and free your hands for other critical tasks like fighting, climbing, or texting.

Critical Point: No Matter What Bandage You Have, Stuff It Within an Actively Bleeding Wound Rather than Just Laying It on Top

In the military doctrine of TCCC, once the casualty and care providers are out of immediate danger from further injury, then more calculated decisions may be made in the Tactical Field Care phase of care. The most critical principle continues to be controlling hemorrhage. Thus, if a wound is still bleeding externally, the situation needs to be escalated, and something more needs to be done. This may involve any or all of the abovementioned techniques and largely depends on the anatomy of the wound. Conversely, a secondary principle remains minimizing unnecessary pain and morbidity. Effective tourniquets induce profound limb ischemia within minutes which is extremely painful, as well as completely distracting from any task. Thus, if the casualty is NOT in shock and it is possible for a diligent care provider to observe for rebleeding, it is preferable to convert tourniquets to either pressure dressings or hemostatic dressings contained with a wound clamp(s). The TCCC recommends that every effort be made to convert tourniquets to some other hemorrhage controls modality within 2 h of tourniquet application.

Extreme Environments

The use of the term "extreme environment" is NOT meant as any disservice to the sacrifices of our Armed Forces personnel, as facing oncoming combatants with a traumatically amputated extremity or coughing up blood from multiple torso wounds should fit the definition of extreme in anybody's understanding. The term is therefore used to communicate novel environments in which human physiology is functioning at the limit of sustainable, and any further degradation through hemorrhage has an extreme risk of crossing the line into unsustainable anaerobic acid producing dysoxia and irreversible cumulative oxygen debt. Within the death zone on Mount Everest, oxygen saturation is already only marginally supportive of life. Loss of even minimal oxygen-carrying capacity would likely be fatal, and thus, the key is not how to control hemorrhage but how quickly it is achieved. This really is a tactical situation in which the Mountain will quickly win unless blood loss is immediately quelled. Therefore, the recommendations would mirror those in a tactical scenario emphasizing immediate self-aid with direct pressure. Unfortunately holding direct pressure while trying to descend Mount Everest is illusionary, and some follow-on maneuver will be required. This again will be completely dictated by preplanning and what you have brought. Ideally this will be some kind of wound packing sealed with a wound clamp with a dressing if limb function can be preserved or a tourniquet if required, as "descending the death zone of Everest with a tourniquet on any limb" is an oxymoron.

Another so-called extreme environment is space. This environment has multiple definitions that consider threshold barriers to human survival. More specifically, the most practical definition is the altitude of approximately 18 km (60,000 ft) to 19 km (62,000 ft) where water boils at the normal temperature of the human body due to the greatly diminished atmospheric pressure (0.0618 atmosphere or 6.3 kPa (47 mmHg)). In this unpressurized environment, humans die immediately. In order to combat this ultimate challenging environment, the most advanced technology of our species has been compartmentalized into a survival habitat. Although our most advanced hemorrhage control capabilities could be pre-positioned in these environments (e.g., Mars), every ounce of weight must be justified based on a simple probabilistic calculation:

Fig. 20.2 Use any
practical means necessary
to *stop the bleeding!*

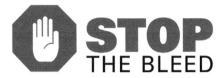

is the astronaut more likely to bleed or starve to death on a 4-year mission to Mars? Depending on the spacecraft design, an astronaut may have the assistance of an ultrasound-guided autonomous surgical robot capable of percutaneously injecting hemostatic foam for torso wounds or autonomously compressing or even stenting peripheral wounds. However, given realistic limitations of mass, volume, and power, the more likely scenario is that an exploration-class space mission will be extremely austere, and astronauts will essentially practice tactical care under fire. The physiology of astronauts within these environments is also unique, as extended duration space missions lead to physiologic responses such as reduction in both the blood volume and the homeostatic responses to blood loss. In other words, if bleeding astronauts do not immediately control the bleeding themselves with manual compression and some wound dressing, they will have lost critical blood volume which will affect them much more profoundly than similar volumes on earth.

Conclusions

Use any practical means necessary to *stop the bleeding!* (Fig. 20.2)

Take-Home Points
1. The first requirement in a firefight is to maintain effective counterfire.
2. As soon as safe, casualties should be moved behind cover especially if auto-care is required.
3. If no external care can be expected, casualties must assess and care for themselves.
4. A tourniquet is an effective hemorrhage control device for extremity wounds but will completely incapacitate that extremity.
5. A wound clamp is an alternate extremity hemorrhage control device that may not be as effective as a tourniquet if not used in conjunction with wound packing but it typically does not incapacitate a limb.

The pleasure of a physician is little, the gratitude of patients is rare, and even rarer is material reward, but these things will never deter the student who feels the call within him/her.
Theodor Billroth

Further Reading

1. St John AE, Wang X, Lim EB, Chien D, Stern SA, White NJ. Effects of rapid wound sealing on survival and blood loss in a swine model of lethal junctional arterial hemorrhage. J Trauma Acute Care Surg. 2015;79(2):256–62. doi:10.1097/TA.0000000000000746.

Chapter 21
Hemorrhage in the Critical Care Environment: Do We Have to Go Back to the OR?

Neil G. Parry and Morad Hameed

Case Scenario

A morbidly obese 66-year-old female has been admitted to your intensive care unit for 21 days following a neurologic insult. The nurse interrupts your rounds to notify you that the patient has copious amounts of blood pouring out of her tracheostomy and is grossly unstable…

Patients in the intensive care unit (ICU) are by definition complex, are usually very ill, and can be some of the most demanding patients within our practices to manage. They are often in multi-organ failure, hemodynamically unstable, on vasopressors, and/or mechanically ventilated. There may be multiple, often conflicting reasons to account for their tachycardia or hypotension. As such, their physiologic response to bleeding may not be as obvious as one would expect. It will also certainly be more challenging to diagnose.

Having said that, any change in clinical and physiologic status of an ICU patient mandates immediate and thorough evaluation. Bleeding should always be in the differential, and like many things in surgery, we need to rapidly identify or exclude the most serious threats to life.

Look for Surgical Bleeding!!!

Surgical bleeding needs to be identified and treated aggressively with definitive surgery or with some interventional procedure. If you are not a surgeon, call one!

N.G. Parry, MD, FRCSC, FACS
General Surgery, Trauma and Critical Care, Departments of Surgery and Medicine, Schulich School of Medicine, Western University, London, ON, Canada

M. Hameed, MD, MPH, FRCSC, FACS (✉)
Department of Surgery, University of British Columbia, Vancouver, BC, Canada
e-mail: morad.hameed@vch.ca

© Springer International Publishing AG 2018
C.G. Ball, E. Dixon (eds.), *Treatment of Ongoing Hemorrhage*,
DOI 10.1007/978-3-319-63495-1_21

At the bedside, look for obvious bleeding. Check surgical sites, all orifices, and for that matter the bed. Check all tubes (nasogastric tube, chest tubes, urinary catheter, or surgical drains). Evaluate all body cavities for fluid which can be readily done with clinical examination and point of care ultrasound.

Once a bleeding source has been identified, interventions include transfusion of warmed blood products (and possible massive transfusion protocol), correction of coagulopathies, and source control. ICU patients, thankfully, generally have excellent IV access, and although painfully obvious, early surgical consultation is essential.

Once source control has been identified, follow protocols from earlier chapters for surgical control. The more common sources of major bleeding in the ICU include traumatic hemorrhage, postoperative surgical bleeding, gastrointestinal (usually upper), and coagulopathy induced.

There are however a few bleeding situations that are unique to the ICU.

Beware of Hemoptysis with the "Big Yellow Snake"

The pulmonary artery catheter (PAC) was once ubiquitous in ICUs across the globe and is now used very selectively (thankfully!). One of the feared but rare complications associated with its use is pulmonary artery (PA) rupture secondary to either perforation from the PAC tip or, more commonly, from the balloon overdistension. Any hemoptysis or new pleural effusion in a patient with a PAC requires immediate evaluation for a possible PA rupture.

Initial management includes definitive airway management with oral tracheal intubation (if not already intubated) and placing the patient in the lateral decubitus position with the affected, bleeding side down (same side as the tip of the PAC!). Resuscitation with blood products and reversal of any coagulopathy are essential. This is *not* the time to insert a double-lumen endotracheal tube. Bronchoscopy and occlusion of affected side with balloon tamponade are very helpful. This is accomplished by passing a Fogarty catheter down beside (and outside) the endotracheal tube under bronchoscopic guidance. Overinflating the balloon or increasing the positive end-expiratory pressure (PEEP) can be attempted but has had mixed results with slowing down the hemorrhage.

Most patients with large-volume hemoptysis and a new pleural effusion should be emergently taken to the operating theater where definitive surgical intervention may occur. This would include a thoracotomy on the affected side followed by hilar clamping with repair or ligation of PA and/or its branch, lobectomy or even pneumonectomy. Patients with small-volume hemoptysis who are relatively more stable should be taken to angiography for transcatheter embolization of their pseudoaneurysm.

Minor Bleed with Tracheostomy May Not Be So Minor

Bleeding in the first 48 h after tracheostomy insertion (percutaneous or open) is usually venous and may be controlled with local measures such as pressure, sutures, or topical hemostatic agents.

Bleeding several weeks later is much more worrisome and may be due to a trachea-innominate fistula. Of course, the best way to treat this awful complication is with prevention. Prior to performing a percutaneous tracheostomy in the ICU, always look and palpate for abnormal pulsation in the sternoclavicular notch. Be sure to place the tracheostomy in the first or second tracheal ring and never go down too low.

Any minor bleeding around the tracheostomy site or within the ventilator circuit should be investigated with bronchoscopy to localize the source. In cases of massive bleeding, and suspected trachea-innominate fistula, the immediate goals are to control the airway and tamponade the bleeding. In the patient that has a non-cuffed tube, one must either replace it with a cuffed tracheostomy (over a tube exchanger) or an oral endotracheal tube. Bleeding can be often controlled by simply overinflating the cuff. This will buy you precious time to get to the operating room (OR). However, if this is not successful, extend the incision around the tracheostomy and bluntly dissect the pretracheal space inferiorly. Then, hook your finger anteriorly up against the sternum to tamponade the innominate artery. This is best accomplished with oral endotracheal intubation but can be done with the tracheostomy in situ if the tracheostomy incision is extended inferiorly.

Of course, any coagulopathy must be corrected and a massive transfusion protocol should be initiated. The arterial line should be on the left as the innominate artery will be ligated at some point if you can successfully get the patient to the OR. Once in the OR, a median sternotomy is performed, and the innominate vein should be retracted inferiorly (or transected) for better exposure of the innominate artery. The innominate artery can then be ligated proximal and distal to the arterial defect. Reconstruction incurs a much higher risk of bleeding and is not necessary as the risk of stroke is low. Primary repair is generally not feasible because of excessive tension once the defect has been debrided back to healthy tissue. The tracheal injury, however, can be repaired primarily once the edges have been debrided, and a tissue interposition with either muscle (sternocleidomastoid or strap muscles) or thymus should be placed between the ligated artery and tracheal defect. Endovascular stents in the innominate artery have also been described to arrest the acute hemorrhage.

Dreaded Coagulopathies

The acute traumatic coagulopathy of trauma, also known as trauma-induced coagulopathy, is a complex process that involves the disruption of anticoagulant factors, procoagulant factors, endothelial activation, fibrinolysis, and platelet dysfunction; it is *not* simply a dilutional or consumptive coagulopathy. It occurs very early after major traumatic injury and is quite common (up to 25%). This coagulopathy is worsened with the accompanying acidemia and hypothermia often seen in the multiple injured patient. Just as its pathophysiology is complex, so is its management.

Early detection is key but difficult. Many centers promote the use of viscoelastic assays (such as thromboelastography or thromboelastometry) to test the clotting efficiency and guide blood product resuscitation. Others employ balanced resuscitation with massive transfusion protocols (e.g., 1:1:1 PRBC/FFP/platelets with tranexamic acid) and early use of plasma. Regardless, bleeding patients do not need crystalloids; they need blood products. Patients must be kept warm with warmed blood products and blankets (preferably, forced hot air blankets, e.g., Bair Hugger). Adequate perfusion must be ensured to decrease the acidemia, and rapid control of surgical bleeding is essential. Target blood pressure goal of 80–90 mmHg systolic is adequate if there is a correctible bleeding source (i.e., controlled by surgery or endoluminal procedure) and no traumatic brain injury.

Medical coagulopathies are another matter unto themselves. Disseminated intravascular coagulopathy (DIC) is caused by disruption of both activation and regulation of multiple coagulation pathways. This can lead to thrombin generation which can cause organ failure as well as consumption of coagulation factors and platelets which may cause diffuse bleeding. Unfortunately, there is not one magic laboratory test to diagnosis DIC. It is a dynamic process, and the diagnosis should be made on both clinical and laboratory information. The mainstay in managing DIC is to treat the underlying cause.

However, all efforts should be made to reverse the coagulopathy with patients in DIC who are at high risk of bleeding or who are clinically bleeding. Platelets should be transfused if less than 50×10^9/L; elevated INR (>1.5 times normal) should be reversed with transfusion of fresh frozen plasma. Prothrombin complex concentrates may be used if the patient is fluid overloaded but they will not fully correct the deficit. Cryoprecipitate should be transfused if fibrinogen is less than 1 g/L. However, abnormal laboratory values *without* active bleeding or significant risk of bleeding should not be aggressively treated.

Thrombocytopenia, on its own, is fairly common in the ICU and results from decreased production, increased destruction, or increased consumption of platelets. Once again, there are multiple underlying causes (e.g., sepsis, drug induced, immunologic, hypersplenism, to name a few), and treating them will often normalize the platelet counts. As previously mentioned, patients with platelet counts <50×10^9/L that are bleeding or at high risk of bleeding should be transfused, and those not at risk of bleeding should be transfused when platelet counts <10×10^9/L to prevent a major bleeding episode (specifically intracranial).

Liver failure and renal failure also pose specific challenges to the bleeding patient. Most hemostatic proteins are produced in the liver, and reduced synthesis results in prolonged bleeding times, reduced platelet counts (direct result from alcohol), and increased fibrinolytic activity. Cholestatic liver disease decreases absorption of lipid soluble factors II, VII, IX, and X, thereby reducing the amount of vitamin K. Uremic patients have dysfunctional platelets and von Willebrand factor.

Apart from blood component therapy, when these patients bleed, they may benefit from desmopressin and conjugated estrogens (to improve platelet function), erythropoietin (renal), and tranexamic acid (more for renal again).

Bleeding is common in the ICU. Patients are challenging, may have very little physiologic reserve, and, therefore, require aggressive investigation and management.

Take-Home Points
1. ICU patients are complex and significant bleeding may not always be obvious.
2. All bleeding should initially be considered surgical until proven otherwise.
3. Beware of the herald bleed in patients with a pulmonary artery catheter and/or a tracheostomy.
4. Traumatic coagulopathy is inherently different than medical coagulopathy.
5. Viscoelastic assays and massive transfusion protocols are often used for traumatic bleeding.
6. Medical coagulopathies should be aggressively reversed in patients at high risk of bleeding or who are actively bleeding.

Treat every patient like he was a member of your family. David V. Feliciano

Index

© Springer International Publishing AG 2018
C.G. Ball, E. Dixon (eds.), *Treatment of Ongoing Hemorrhage*,
DOI 10.1007/978-3-319-63495-1

Printed in the United States
By Bookmasters